The Salts of the Earth and Synthetic Insanity

The Salts of the Earth and Synthetic Insanity

The Bipolar Theory: A Physical Explanation of Bipolar Mental Illness

Dennis Miller, R.Ph.

iUniverse, Inc.
New York Lincoln Shanghai

The Salts of the Earth and Synthetic Insanity
The Bipolar Theory: A Physical Explanation of Bipolar Mental Illness

iUniverse, Inc.

For information address:
iUniverse, Inc.
2021 Pine Lake Road, Suite 100
Lincoln, NE 68512
www.iuniverse.com

ISBN: 0-595-31499-6 (Pbk)
ISBN: 0-595-66325-7 (Cloth)

Printed in the United States of America

CONTENTS

ACKNOWLEDGEMENTS

I want to thank God, my wife, and my children. You made this book possible. I want to thank Alice for believing in me. I really needed that support. I want to thank Paula for reading my email. I want to thank Hayne for your kindness, dedication, and understanding. I want to thank the sweet ladies in the shop on Gold Hill Road for having the right ingredients. I want to thank Dee and Donna for your service in a critical time. I want to thank the rest of my extended family for loving me, even in difficult circumstances. I am sure others would have left me abandoned. I want to thank my Mother for giving me the belief as a child that I could accomplish anything with hard work and perseverance. I want thank my Dad, God rest his soul, for always being there for me.

Preface

This book should be used in coordination with your doctor in the hope that better therapy will be the outcome. It is important to recognize that you should not do this alone. Like with most things, inappropriate use can have significant consequences. Human physiology relies on balance. Your physician is in the best position to help your achieve the vitamin and mineral balance required for success in this therapy.

I have written this book to quicken the pace of research. I believe my findings are true and correct. I believe the answers are now at our fingertips and the gifted and dedicated people of science can verify them. Over the last 8 months, I have become familiar with only a few researchers' work. I am astonished at the amount of effort these researchers put forth, for little pay or recognition. They are truly the stars of the academic universe. There just may be a new world that awaits us. A world without bipolar disease would be a very different world.

INTRODUCTION

As for my credentials, I do have a bachelors of Science degree in pharmacy. I am not a physician. I am not a laboratory medical researcher. This is even my first book and I do not anticipate a second. I guess my best credential is that I have a little knowledge, I am bipolar and I am the father of a bipolar son. I am also a man who has gone from spending 400 dollars each month on prescription medicine down to zero with the blessing of his psychiatrist of 14 years. That is a validation that transcends professional titles and honors. This is I knew I had established my credibility when my doctor, impressed with my appearance, wanted to know my therapeutic regimen. My credibility is based on results. In the twenties, a young unknown patent clerk in Germany wrote a book that changed the world. He was bipolar too. I am certain that I am not in Einstein's intelligence category; but, like him, I am an unknown looking in the right direction. I believe I have proven that this condition is a kidney disease, not a brain disorder. I am not an expert in kidney disease or liver disease or the endocrine system, but I now have a working knowledge of each. I hope physicians with these specialties will take some time to test my theory. My internet sources are impeccable. Virtually all of my internet research sources are from major universities, medical journals, or the National Institute of Health. During these nine months, I was a detective who would follow the paths led by the physical clues. My hope is that this is a significant work that will lead to the betterment of humanity.

The importance of this discovery is not only for today, but also for the future. I am certain we can now identify children at a very early age and we can get them the treatment necessary for them to live healthy fulfilled and intelligent lives. It is estimated that 1 percent of the population has this disease. However, I believe that this estimation is low. This disease to a greater extent affects many more. However, even at 1% the numbers become staggering. This means that 3 million people in the United States have bipolar disease. That is a lot of sadness and failure.

As most people know bipolar disease or manic depression is a disease where there is considerable fluctuation in mood. A person with this disease may experience days of utter euphoria, "life couldn't get any better", but mostly there are days of "just trying to get by." Anxiety and foreboding fills those days.

A quick temper is very common. There may be insomnia and "sleeping in". Personal hygiene may be poor. This person may actually feel they are trying harder than anyone else, yet nothing gets done. In academics, they may be the brightest in one class and extremely deficient in others. Einstein is a great example. He obviously was a genius in math, but he was a failure in language arts. As much as he worked with speed in relationship to the universe, he could not drive a car. Bipolar people tend to be perfectionists who face their worst enemy in the mirror every day. This disease can lead to disaster in personal relationships as they "wear out" friends with their "Dr. Jekyll and Mr. Hyde" personality. A person whose moods are very stable and happy would never understand the torment that a person with this disease must bear.

It is important to understand that just as for "normal" people those members of the bipolar community, even with this treatment, may need additional help from psychologists and the ministry. They may also need medicine from time to time during periods of crisis just like anyone else. The explanation in this book does not solve the problem, but it does explain it so we can understand what is happening. I believe knowing what is happening is the first step to resolution.

I developed a list of physical complaints I experienced as a person with bipolar disease. I believe this table is unique. I have never seen a comprehensive list of physical symptoms for bipolar disease.

Table 1 <u>Physical Complaints of Bipolar Patients</u>
  Warm skin=zinc and bicarbonate
  Memory= magnesium and acetylcholine
  Mood=magnesium and manganese
  Balance=magnesium
  Belching=excessive chlorine
  Explosive diarrhea=excessive chlorine
  Alternately extreme constipation=magnesium deficiency
  Hot skin=zinc
  Flatulence=excessive chlorine
  Polyphagia (excessive eating)=phosphate deficiency
  Perspiration=excessive sodium and potassium exchange
  Tremors=copper
  Sleep excessively=manganese deficiency
  Sweaty palms=zinc
  Excitability=excessive chlorine
  Lethargy=iron deficiency anemia and/or phosphate deficiency
  Runny nose=possibly parathyroid, pituitary

Amblyopia=possibly, from phosphate deficiency at time of formation

Dilated pupils=magnesium and acetylcholine

Afternoon swoon=chromium and manganese

Hunger or sweet craving =phospho-fructokinase deficiency. A decrease in ATP

probably produces a request for glucose or deficient bicarbonate

Possibly acne from bromine reabsorption in acidosis.*

Night blindness=zinc and vitamin A

Increased bleed times= manganese (vitamin K)

Soft or raspy voice=hyperparathyroidism[1] or phosphate deficiency

Right eye pain aka migraine=possibly hyperparathyroidism

Right kidney awareness=hydroxylase failure

Anger=inversely proportional to buffering capacity, in theory

(I have seen evidence that may suggest that as the acid-base system neutralizes bromine excretion may occur producing a decrease in acne).

In families with a prior history of the disease, the **absence of scalp hair in newborns** provides initial diagnostic evidence for HVDRR[2] (HVDRR stands for 1,25 dihydroxyvitamin D resistant rickets). If you have a bald baby with colic chances are he may have this disease.

Commonly observed symptoms of mania include:

- Normally amiable people may become increasingly angry, impulsive, emotional or irritable
- Intense *euphoria* that nothing can disturb, but if their plans are foiled they may become irritable or uncontrollably furious
- A few manics may become *paranoid or violent* and assault others verbally or physically
- Very *rapid speech*, incessant and usually in a loud voice
- Unable to sleep or sit still…often going for days with 2 or3 hrs sleep and not feeling tired
- *Socially frenetic*…throwing parties, going to bars

[1] http://www.contemporarysurgery.com/11_02/1102Hypp.pdf
[2] http://edrv.endojournals.org/cgi/content/full/20/2/156

- Throw aside normal inhibitions and become sexually hyperactive or promiscuous
- Due to impaired judgment very *poor decision making* skills. Overspending, over commitment, quitting jobs, etc.

Suicidal behaviors may include:

- Extreme personality changes
- Loss of interest in activities that used to be enjoyable
- Significant loss or gain in appetite
- Difficulty falling asleep or wanting to sleep all day
- Fatigue or loss of energy
- Feelings of worthlessness or guilt
- Withdrawal from family and friends
- Neglect of personal appearance or hygiene
- Sadness, irritability, or indifference
- Drug or alcohol use or abuse
- Aggressive, destructive, or defiant behavior
- Poor school performance
- Hallucinations or unusual beliefs[3]

The basis of my theory relief on vitamin pathway failure. The cause of this failure involves losses of minerals that are needed for catalyzing vitamin reactions and phosphate deficiency which is also necessary for vitamin performance. The vitamins affected by this disorder are what I call the "big three." The big three include the water-soluble vitamins thiamine, pyridoxine, and ascorbic acid (vitamin B1, vitamin B6, and vitamin C, respectively).

Hallmark signs of thiamine deficiency include fatigue, irritation, poor memory, mania and depression (confabulation), stocking glove cyanosis, sweating, warm skin, and carbohydrate cravings. Note that these coincide with those of bipolar disease.

Vitamin B6 synthesizes tryptophan to serotonin and is metabolized to niacin in the process. Vitamin B6 is involved in the synthesis of dopamine, NE, and GABA. Vitamin B6 is involved in hemoglobin production. Vitamin B6 may decrease the effect of steroid hormones by binding steroid receptor sites. *Vitamin B6 deficiency produces irritability, depression, confusion, mouth ulcers, increased*

---

[3] http://namiwi.nami.org/helpline/teensuicide.html

dietary protein causes increased vitamin B6 requirement. Homocysteine, a compound linked to atherosclerosis and stress, conversion is regulated by folic acid, B12, and B6. High doses of vitamin B6 decreases the incidence of kidney stones.

Vitamin C is involved with the immune system. Vitamin C is needed for white cell function. Vitamin C is needed also for energy. It is needed for conversion of lysine to carnitine. Vitamin C is needed for serotonin and melatonin production as well as dopamine and NE production. Vitamin C deficiency may result in sleep disturbances and possibly depression. **Vitamin C is involved in hydroxylase synthesis,** particularly of the amino acids lysine and proline. Copper and vitamin C are involved with lysine hydroxylation in collagen synthesis. **Vitamin C and copper are involved with dopamine beta hydroxylase.**[4]

Folic acid is responsible for one-carbon transfers in purine and pyridine (protein) metabolism. Anemia may result from deficiency. Folic acid is involved in DNA synthesis and the synthesis of S-adenosylmethionine or SAM. SAM has been purported to play a key role in mood.

Today is March 30, eight months since starting this therapy. I went to see my psychiatrist of 14 years. He is an astute man who has learned to read the physical signs of mental illness. In the past 13 years he never, ever mentioned anything positive about my appearance. However, during my last appointment he said, "Continue whatever you are doing because it is working." During this appointment he mentioned the same thing, but this time he wanted to know what I using for treatment. So I gave him a brief synopsis of the therapy listed in Chapter 35. I believe, with all my heart, that this is the avenue we bipolar people should be traveling and he apparently thinks so as well.

I have used a symptom-based scheme to develop this book. I have included sections on discovery, symptoms, physiology, and drug abuse plus suicide. I will discuss each symptom approximately in the order of discovery.

---

[4] aamm.unm.edu/get_pic.php?p_id=213

SECTION 1

PHYSICAL DISCOVERIES

CHAPTER 1

Emergency

Somewhere in the "Twilight Zone"

How do you react as a father, mother, husband or wife when you learn that a loved one has a disease that can kill them? This is a story about love as much as it is science. I was faced with that dilemma and the medicines were not working. I felt compelled to act. So I began to learn.

I was working that night in March when I got the call. For those of you who don't know me I am a pharmacist. You know, the friendly guy behind the counter at the local drugstore in whose hands you entrust your life through the use of the medicines I dispense. It was 9:30 in the evening when my wife called. She was in a state of hysteria. I knew immediately from the sound of her voice what had happened. Our intelligent fun loving pre-pubescent son of two years ago had attempted suicide. After a brief stay at the hospital, he was admitted to an excellent facility in Columbia, SC for treatment. For three weeks he was separated from his family. We were only permitted very brief phone calls and a once a week visitation of 30 minutes. When he returned he was stable, but extremely medicated. It was very hard watching him during this time. My memory would recall the good times, laughter and joy in his voice that was muted by some post-pubertal change. Now, however, that joyous voice was silenced by medication.

I believe bipolar disorder is in a way a developmental type of disease. In other words, as the size of the body and skeleton increases the demands on the kidney function also increases. If this demand cannot be met, then consequences will be incurred. Some children exhibit symptoms of this condition earlier in life and their condition, I expect, is more severe.

It was now June and his condition was not improving. If anything he was getting worse. I had listened to the doctors and we had followed the therapy, but he had hit a therapeutic impasse. At this junction I started to get concerned. I could no longer sit idle. I began searching for clues that may help.

CHAPTER 2

Bipolar Disease

How does Lithium Carbonate work?

Bipolar affective disorder is a mood disorder characterized by mood swings from mania (exaggerated feeling of well-being, stimulation, and grandiosity in which a person can lose touch with reality) to <u>depression</u> (overwhelming feelings of sadness, anxiety, and low self-worth, which can include suicidal thoughts and suicide attempts). [5] Approximately 1 or 2 percent of the population has this disease. In the United States that means anywhere from 3 to 7 million people have this disease. Bipolar people tend to abuse alcohol and drugs. The devastation in real human terms by this disease is enormous. The inability to maintain employment is frequent. Marriages can be disastrous. Families are literally ripped apart due to the destruction from bipolar disease. Many bipolar people decide ultimately that suicide is the only cure.

I was an excellent student in some areas and deficient in others. This is a common characteristic with people with bipolar disease. I have known people with this disease to be considered geniuses in some academic fields and in other fields completely deficient.

I was diagnosed with bipolar disorder over 12 years ago after a bizarre psychotic episode. It took me almost a year to recover to a point where I again felt somewhat normal. At that time this was, and still is, considered a mental illness that produced extreme swings in the mood from major suicidal depression to

---

[5] http://www.swmedicalcenter.com/13003.cfm

mania. Suicide is the final symptom of this heinous disease. Besides a life of ups and downs, plaqued by real daily misery, the end results in many cases at one's own hands. During these years I accepted what I was told about the disease.

Lithium carbonate was the "gold standard" for the treatment of bipolar disease. Kidney disease was just a side effect listed during chronic treatment with this drug. The kidney is the organ responsible for filtering liquid. The kidney keeps what the body needs and discards what the body no longer requires. Somewhere along the line I read that no other lithium salt, except for the carbonate, worked in bipolar treatment. Lithium is a mineral element. I stored this information for later recall. **This investigation provides an explanation for the method of action for lithium carbonate. Lithium produces a parathyroid related hypocalcemia.**[6] The parathyroid is an endocrine gland that regulates calcium metabolism. Until now, the explanation given was simply "unknown." It seemed to me that if no other form of lithium worked, then maybe it was the carbonate and not the lithium that was important. I personally used lithium carbonate for several years, until the very real possibility of permanent kidney damage due to this use forced me to seek other remedies.

Environmental stress can produce profound changes in genetics. I believe this disease is a result of environmental stress. Many centuries ago, the world was covered with potash from volcanic eruptions. Potash contains substantial amounts of phosphorus. I believe bipolar disease is an adaptation due to this environmental stress. A bipolar person with their ability to excrete large amounts of phosphorus and other minerals would stand a much better chance of surviving in this volcanically polluted environment. Even their randy nature would be a good thing to help perpetuate the human race.

---

[6] http://www.emedicine.com/ent/topic539.htm

CHAPTER 3

Bipolar Theory Definition

"I'm not crazy. I'm just a little unwell"
—Matchbox 20

The first question I asked myself was, "What do I know?" That is, "What symptoms am I seeing? The answering of this first question, followed by a multitude of other questions, set me on an Internet journey and back to basic sciences. Back in 1979 after I had graduated from pharmacy school, I purchased the medical text Harrison's Principles of Internal Medicine. Over the years, I had rarely used this text, but it looked nice. Specifically, I will mention Harrison's and The Merck Manual as key resources in identifying this disease pathology.

It wasn't until my son became sick that I began to investigate each individual physical symptom. Initially, I expected a fruitless search, but to my amazement each search yielded fruit until there was a bountiful harvest. With each identified symptom, I found a mineral and a cure for that symptom. After a time of intense research, I reached the conclusion that virtually all cations were being detrimentally affected.

A cation is a mineral with a positive charge. What was causing this cation loss? To my knowledge only (1) ingestion of adequate quantities of minerals, (2) absorption failure through excessive diarrhea, (3) absorption failure from intestinal anatomic malformation or (4) excessive excretion by the kidneys would be factors involving mineral loss. I thought through each pathway. I rejected number one because I usually ate as much or more than most "normal" people. I rejected number two because even though I experienced sporadic episodes of diarrhea they simply were not frequent enough to warrant scrutiny. I rejected number three because in a condition where there are anatomical problems the symptoms appear very early in life. So, that left only number four. The kidneys. The kidneys made sense. The kidney is the king when it comes to filtration of fluids in the body.

All of this investigation leads me to a statement that will certainly cause uproar among many medical professionals, but I feel absolutely compelled to state this theory. Bipolar (manic-depression) illness is NOT a mental illness, but rather a physical disease caused by the *less than optimal* performance of a certain group of enzymes known as hydroxylases. This hydroxylase deficiency produces physical manifestations that result in mineral losses via malabsorption, biliary insufficiency, and excessive urinary excretion. Many vitamin pathway failures, especially thiamine and pyridoxine, occur that result in mental symptoms. Principally, the active form of vitamin D (1,25 dihydroxycholecalciferol) fails to be synthesized in one kidney, or the quantity of active vitamin D is insufficient to meet physical demands, due to a decrease in 1 alpha hydroxylase. (The amount of vitamin D precursors may be excessive due to this synthesis failure, which may lead to symptoms of vitamin D toxicity). The result is increased phosphate excretion, increased bicarbonate excretion, increased chloride ion reabsorption to compensate for phosphate and bicarbonate buffer loss, metabolic acidosis, and respiratory alkalosis. The failure of 7 alpha hydroxylase results in mineral losses, especially of the trace elements, through a down-regulated bile system. Mania occurs from extrarenal synthesis for active vitamin D, which produces increased phosphate levels. Depression occurs from system exhaustion. That was a mouth full. The rest of this book will be organized to prove this theory by examining the physical symptoms of this disease. This book may test average readers knowledge of medical terms. I will do my best to provide a good human analogy to define some common terms, but I suggest an Internet Website like Dorland's or Hyperdictionary to provide the definitions to difficult terms.

An enzyme is a protein that helps speed a chemical reaction. An enzyme can be looked at as a preacher at a wedding. He does not take part in the marriage, but he joins the bride and groom in holy matrimony.

If the reader sees -ase at the end of a word this refers to a specific enzyme. In this case, hydroxylase is an enzyme the body uses to split water into a hydrogen ion and a hydroxide ion. Most people know the chemical formula for water is H_2O. Restating that the formula, H_2O becomes HOH or in ionic terms $H+$ + $OH-$. (A much more in depth analysis will follow in later chapters). If this reaction does not occur, then many other necessary metabolic reactions cannot proceed.

It is important to understand that there are several forms of vitamin D and all have some physical action on the body, but the primary active form of vitamin D is technically called 1,25 dihydroxy cholecalciferol or DHCC for short.

CHAPTER 4

Hyperchloremic Acidosis

Too much bleach in the wash

Bipolar disease affects virtually every physiologic process, but usually mildly. The physical symptoms of this disease are many, and "fly under the radar" of health care professionals because the results of blood tests are "normal". *The cations or positively charged minerals are actually low normal in virtually all categories.* The actual levels of mineral deficiency may be worse than the blood test show, when coupled with the fact that many of these ions are protein bound. When a mineral is said to be protein bound this means that the mineral is physically "glued" to that protein and, therefore, the mineral is not available to react. Protein levels also tend to be low in a person with bipolar disease. The part of the kidney that appears to be affected, the distal renal tubule, only filters about 5 percent of the total fluid, but this small loss over the long term produces a debt that must eventually be paid. In the kidney there are two tubules. The one closest to the glomerulus is known as the proximal renal tubule and the one farthest away is known as the distal renal tubule. The term renal refers to the kidney. Ultimately, this distal renal tubule fails to produce adequate amounts of 1 alpha hydroxylase, an enzyme necessary for calcium and phosphate reabsorption. *This failure results in excessive urinary excretion of calcium and phosphate. The loss of phosphate ion in particular results in excessive amounts of chloride ion being reabsorbed to maintain proper neutral acid-base levels in the body.* It is absolutely imperative that the body maintains this neutrality. The chloride ion helps to achieve neutrality, but at a high cost paid for by adverse effects. *This excessive chloride ion (also known as "anion gap") and acid-base imbalance produces many of the symptoms associated with bipolar illness.* An example of an acid would be something tart like lemon juice. An example of something basic would be baking soda. Chlorine intoxication produces excitability and apprehension (two common symptoms associated with bipolar disease). Researcher Kaye Kilburne found that chlorine intoxication produces balance and memory loss (also common symptoms). [7]

Acidosis is defined as a physiologic disturbance which tends to add acid or remove alkali from body fluids.[8] Metabolic acidosis is caused by one of these mechanisms (1) increased production of non-volatile acids, (2) decreased acid excretion by the kidney, (3) loss of alkali. In intracellular fluid excess protons replace potassium which shifts out of cells, tending to elevate plasma levels. Extracellular bicarbonate is reduced by reaction with hydrogen ion or, in patients wasting alkali, by loss of bicarbonate in urine or stool.[9] Certain sugars used for parenteral admintration, such as fructose, may cause lactic acidosis.[10] Chronic metabolic acidosis is the hallmark of renal tubular acidosis.[11]

Originally when I began researching this condition I hoped to find something that may help my son, but I never expected to find a cure. I truly expected an impenetrable roadblock along the way, but this never happened. Each pathway skillfully fit with the other until this concept just made sense. I have spent over nine months preparing this book and I have poured over thousands of sources before finishing this theory.

My Internet sources basically helped to identify which cations were being lost. I made it a point to choose impeccable sources. You will find that virtually all of my sources are from major universities, medical journals, and the National Institute of Health. Cations are positively charged mineral elements. You might recognize the names calcium, magnesium, potassium, copper, zinc, etc. It is important to understand what happens when an anion gap exists. An anion gap produces too many negative charges and not enough positive charges to produce neutralization.

Much of life is about balance and, physiologically, life cannot exist properly without neutrality or balance. When an anion gap exists then too much hydrogen ion remains in the body and metabolic acidosis occurs. Normally bicarbonate is reabsorbed in the kidney to maintain neutral fluids. (We call this a buffer). There is a mechanism in the body that can move large amounts of acidic bicarbonate ion to neutral hydrogen bicarbonate. This mechanism is called the carbonic anhydrase system and zinc plays a major role in its working. If there is excess hydrogen bicarbonate, then it becomes carbon dioxide. The lungs expire the carbon dioxide. In this disease phosphate ion fails to be reabsorbed so the next more

---

[7] http://www.niih.go.jp/en/indu_hel/2003/pdf/ih_41_4_01.pdf

[8] Harrison's Principles of Internal Medicine, 10th Edition, page 231.

[9] Harrison's Principles of Internal Medicine, 10th Edition, page 232.

[10] Harrison's Principles of Internal Medicine, 10th Edition, page 232.

[11] Harrison's Principles of Internal Medicine, 10th Edition, page 232.

readily available anion is reabsorbed to maintain neutral pH. *Chloride ion does not have the buffering capacity of the carbonic anhydrase system so the body continues to get more acidic.* This additional acid or positive charge is exchanged for other positive ions, calcium, magnesium, potassium, copper, zinc, etc. in the kidney fairly indiscriminately in order to maintain neutrality.

This is where the subtle problems occur. This is an odd combination of mild states of metabolic acidosis and respiratory alkalosis. These positive ions are lost in a slightly higher quantity over a long period of time, which results in a metabolic state that approaches deficiency. The trouble here is that these *minerals are necessary to run rate limited enzymatic reactions* in the body, specifically to catalyze vitamins. These minerals can be looked at as the ring in the wedding we mentioned previously. The ring helps the wedding proceed much more quickly. So, the result is a body that runs very inefficiently. I have mentioned many symptoms of bipolar disease later in this book. Each symptom has a mineral deficiency that has produced the symptom. As each mineral is restored each symptom disappears. Many vitamins have a specific or multiple mineral cofactors necessary for that vitamin to do its work. *With low amounts of minerals present in the body, metabolism does still occur but at a much slower rate and with less production.*

So what you get is what I call the bipolar man. **He is a tired, candy or alcohol craving insomniac with a runny nose and dilated eyes. He needs contacts or eyeglasses. He may appear angry or he may have an unpleasant disposition. Importantly, he has some type of rickets-like defect of scoliosis, sunken chest, knock-kneed, dental defects, etc.**

After having lived with the disease for 47 years I had accepted its fate and I was regulated with expensive medicines prescribed by my doctor. I would take my Trileptal before work and my Effexor at bedtime with my clonazepam for sleep, day in and day out. Mindlessly accepting what the medical establishment had given me. I had lived with the torment that bipolar disease brings.

I believe probably nothing in the life of a normal person could conceivably describe the day in day out torment that a person with uncontrolled bipolar disease has. This is a devastating disease that eventually takes away a person's will to live. This disease is a killer, undeniably. Society has little sympathy for a person with this condition. Rather than have empathy for this person, society in general labels that person as lazy, belligerent, ill tempered, and dirty. Rather than inclusion, society excludes them as outcasts. They become the friendless loner. Now the time has come for the loner to take his place in society. I believe that this disease can be diagnosed very early in life and that this life can proceed "normally."

CHAPTER 5

Warm Skin

"Joe Cool"—The first discovery, zinc

This chapter and further chapters involve a lot of discussion involving chemistry. In order to make this more understandable try imagining you are a cashier and the object of your work is to make change to complete the transaction. Imagine the ions we will be talking about are dollar bills and quarters, dimes, nickels and pennies. If you are a cashier and you are low on cash and someone hands you a hundred dollar bill you will not be able to make change and your customer may get upset, but if your cash register has plenty of cash making change and completing the transaction is easy even when multiple transactions requiring large bills. The same thing happens in the body. In order for most vitamins to work a catalyst, also known as a cofactor, must be present. In the normal body the cofactor and the vitamin are both readily available so the reaction occurs and "change is made". However, in the bipolar body "the manager of the store keeps taking all of the twenty dollar bills so making change for a hundred becomes very difficult." That is, something has caused the loss of the cofactor so that the vitamin cannot perform the metabolic reactions necessary for normal life. To make change, a cashier may have to use a combination of currency. For example, to give back $8.11 the cashier needs a 5-dollar bill, 3 one-dollar bills, a dime, and a penny to efficiently provide change. Other combinations can be used but they are less efficient. Therefore, all of these items must be found in the till for peak efficiency to occur. If they are not there, then the transaction does not proceed as efficiently and possibly not at all. The waiting line backs up and the anxious customer says, "Hey, what is taking so long?" However, when the line backs up in the body the excess chemical "waiting in line" usually produces adverse effects.

So if the reader can keep this mental image of the reactions in the body proceeding much like a cashier acting as a catalyst and the money in the till as the ions and protein in the body this information becomes much easier to read.

I experienced the **sweaty palms** on occasion (an important symptom of impending acidosis). I experienced the runny nose and the embarrassment that went with it. I had the gas and the explosive diarrhea. Yes, I too have had the short temper and the anger. I have experienced the hypomania and it's wonderful exhilarating effects. All the while knowing that it was to be short-lived with illness and depression as the eventual result. I knew my changing behaviors made it difficult for people to befriend me. However, I could not change who I was. I was shy and isolated much of the time.

However, when my son was affected severely and I could continue to see his deterioration, even with medication, I felt compelled to learn more about this disease. I wanted to find something or some things that could improve his condition.

I began keeping notes when success occurred. These notes were eventually put on poster board. I would follow one pathway into another into another. Never in this research did a wall of stone halt me. I had really expected a roadblock to appear somewhere since I had never done medical research before this time.

The first symptom I listed was heat. My son's body was warm to the touch. This was a key symptom. *I relearned that energy was produced from the body's use of phosphate.*[12] Some authors go so far as to state that life is defined as the ability to make and break phosphate bonds. This may have something to do with the expression "a fire in your belly." Phosphorus, remember, is the stuff of which matches are made. When you think of phosphorus think of energy.

Before starting this therapy I found it difficult to cuddle for any length of time with my wife because it quickly got too hot. She used to love it on a cold winter night because as she said, "you feel like a heater". *Now we can cuddle for extended periods of time without getting overheated.*

Phosphate is a molecule found in foodstuffs. Phosphate is composed of phosphorus and oxygen. It is phosphate that runs our bodies. Without phosphate we have no energy. Our body's phosphate is carried around on a molecule known as adenosine. It is the cleaving of the phosphate ion from adenosine that provides heat and energy for our body. Those in academics refer to this molecule as ATP meaning adenosine triphosphate. This means there are 3 phosphate ions attached to this molecule. This means three phosphate ions can be given up if needed for

---

[12] http://www.lpi.oregonstate.edu/infocenter/minerals.html

each available adenosine molecule. Obviously, a heated body is a body performing at a high metabolic rate and it uses a lot of phosphate.

A symptom of thiamine deficiency or beriberi is **warm skin.** I made an assumption that heat is related to acidity. Acidity is directly related to hydrogen ion. I looked up acidosis in <u>Harrison's</u>, the medical text. I found that acidosis, the formation of too much acid in the body, is controlled by a simple chemical reaction where hydrogen ion and bicarbonate ion are converted back and forth to water and carbon dioxide. This system helps the body maintain strict pH levels of around 7.4. (The chemistry term pH describes the quantity of hydrogen ions in a solution. The pH scale goes from 1 to 14. Seven is considered neutral for chemical reactions. Human physiology requires a slightly basic 7.4pH). If the body is unable to proceed with this reaction, then the body becomes too acidic. I noticed in my research that this reaction was rate limited. I knew from my organic chemistry lessons that rate limited reactions are controlled by catalysts. That is, the chemical reaction will only proceed very slowly unless another ingredient is added to the mix that stimulates the reaction. Usually that catalytic ingredient is a metal or mineral.

In order to simplify things for better understanding I will use the analogy of baking a cake. You must have the eggs, milk, sugar, and flour as ingredients in order to bake a cake. So it is for the human body, it requires vitamins to perform the necessary reactions, catalysts in the form of positively charged minerals, and negatively charged phosphate. Without these ingredients the cake falls flat and so does the human body.

So I embarked on a journey to find the catalyst for this "carbonic reaction". I found that zinc was the necessary ingredient to catalyze this reaction. Also, it made sense that by adding bicarbonate directly to the formula that the reaction would be pushed more toward the water and carbon dioxide side of the equation which would make the body more neutral, not acidic.

So **I gave my son zinc and sodium bicarbonate and his body cooled and he slept.** This was exciting. I had never experienced such a dramatic success.

Upon further research I found that zinc is important in preventing diseases like colds. It is important for our immune system. Zinc is involved in growth and sexual maturation. Zinc is involved in over 100 metabolic reactions. Large concentrations of zinc are found in the eyes. My son had frequent colds and his vision was poor.

Chapter 6

Insomnia and Tremors

"Sleepless in Seattle"

I had lived with the **insomnia**. The night after night of praying I could fall asleep. Wondering if I would ever fall a sleep. I would lie awake and wonder what the new day's consequences would bring if I didn't fall asleep. I would drag myself out of bed and show up, usually late, for work. I was incredibly tired. The afternoon would produce a swoon that would leave me half asleep. People viewed me differently and probably for good reason. I frequently had colds especially after a brief period of feeling good. This is a condition known as hypomania. I was eating candy bars, skipping meals and drinking coffee frequently. I could never please myself with any accomplishment. I simply was never good enough. Finally, the breaking point happened.

After another sleepless night, I got out of bed, my head throbbing, and I readied for work. (The brain, from a news article I read long ago, after significant sleep deprivation produces a substance similar to LSD, the hallucinogen). I made it to the store where I worked. My diet now consisted of candy, cola, and more candy. Sometime around 11 in the morning I received a phone call that I totally misinterpreted. I interpreted the message as "someone kidnapped my children." After a bizarre sequence of events I ended up at the hospital. Upon entering the psych ward I was hooked up to an I.V. I would guess the I.V. was D5W, NS. (This would be normal procedure for a person experiencing dehydration). This is a solution of 5% dextrose, a sugar, water, and normal saline (table salt). I quickly became psychotic.

I believe the sugar and salt finally pushed my fragile body completely "over the edge". I spent the next year of my life recovering to a point where I could function approximately normal. I received haloperidol, a major tranquilizer, for a considerable time after exiting the hospital. This drug basically turns a person into a zombie. I did not feel emotion. There was no love, hate, happiness or sadness. Nothing. The positive side to this drug is it stops thought. I did not think. I merely existed. In many ways I became a vegetable. However, this period gave my brain and body some time to recuperate from the damage it had suffered.

I cannot imagine the combination of emotions that my wife experienced during this time. For some reason she stood beside me. She endured and persevered. Without her, I do not believe this book would have been written. Life does throw "chin music" at you from time to time. I admire her ability to dust her pants off and look for the next pitch.

I had used benzodiazepines, anti-anxiety tablets, over the years to induce sleep. No normal person could understand the fear that nighttime brings to a person with this disease. Without medicine to induce sleep, I knew a long night of movie videos certainly awaited. The routine became "take a pill" and, "aah" sleep. However, the problem with sleeping pills was awakening. These drugs generally cause a "hangover" effect. As a matter of fact, these medicines have been called "freeze dried alcohol," for good reason. Alcohol and benzodiazepines both affect the same neurotransmitter, GABA. A simple analogy of a neurotransmitter is electricity and electrical appliances. These appliances all use electricity, but each appliance may perform a different function like lighting, computing, heating, etc.

William Shakespeare may have, like a lot of writers, had this disease. He certainly understood the nature of insomnia in his writing. Bipolar disease is so common amongst great writers that it almost seems like this disease is a pre-requisite.

In his guilt Mac Beth, like his troubled wife, cannot find the "Sleep that knits up the ravell'd sleeve of care." In "Henry IV," the restless king recognizes the emotional roots of his sleeplessness when he reports "Uneasy lays the head that wears a crown." The study authors agree with Shakespeare that an excess of worry "may produce a hyperarousal that prevents a person from falling asleep." [13]

Sometime during this research I discovered copper and thiamine for sleep induction. This is NOT the same red penny copper, but the green type. **Copper and thiamine convert tryptophan to melatonin, which induces sleep.** A much more involved explanation of this pathway will follow later. This was a wonderful discovery. I no longer needed a prescription drug for sleep during normal stress

---

[13] http://www.personalmd.com/news/a1997102704.shtml

times. I realized that in times of extreme stress that the drug may be necessary, just as it may be required for any normal person. Now, under normal everyday circumstances, I could sleep a full eight hours and awaken feeling rested. Today, on rare sleepless nights, I may additionally use ¼ tablet of an over-the-counter sleeping medicine called melatonin. It is commonly found in a 3mg tablet.

Serotonin, another neurotransmitter, is also derived from tryptophan. Serotonin is the substance that many antidepressants enhance. These drugs make up the class of antidepressants known as SSRI's.

Serotonin is an **indolamine** monoamine neurotransmitter. The synthetic pathway is analogous to the catecholamines in many ways. An important distinction is that the rate-limiting step is the uptake of tryptophan into the neuron. **Tryptophan availability is the actual rate-limiting factor in the intact animal.** Tryptophan crosses the blood brain barrier via an *active transport mechanism* in competition with other neutral amino acids such as leucine, lysine, and methionine. The activity of this transport mechanism is **facilitated by** the presence of **insulin and glucose.** Another interesting aspect of this system is the fact that **tryptophan is** one of the few amino acids which is **bound in the plasma** to any significant degree. The actual **binding site is the fatty acid binding site of the albumen.** This system allows a multitude of factors to ultimately influence the rate-limiting step in serotonin synthesis. For example anything which increases free fatty acids would displace the tryptophan and thus increase the percent free which is able to cross the BBB. Examples of such events include any acute stressor, which increases glucocorticoid response, exercise, and acute alcohol consumption.13

Melatonin, the main hormone produced by the pineal gland, displays a circadian rhythm peaking at night (1). Pinealocytes uses tryptophan as substrate for melatonin synthesis, and melatonin levels change as a function of tryptophan availability (2). Pyridoxine is converted to its active coenzyme form, pyridoxal phosphate (PLP). More than 60 PLP-dependent enzymes are known, including enzymes that participate in decarboxylation reactions such as the decarboxylation of DOPA to dopamine and 5-hydroxytryptophan to serotonin (3-4). The activity of pyridoxine as a coenzyme in the tryptophan metabolism was described in the kinurenine and methoxyindole pathways (5). Pyridoxines act as a coenzyme of 5-hydroxytryptophan decarboxylases. The enzyme performs carboxylation of 5-hydroxytryptophan to serotonin, which is the immediate precursor of melatonin (5). The effect of pyridoxine on aromatic amino acid decarboxylase activity supports a regulatory role of pyridoxine on the synthesis of neurotransmitters (6-7). Melatonin was shown to increase brain pyridoxal phosphokinase activity, inhibition of glutaminergic neurotransmission, resulting in inhibitory effects on central nervous system activity (8). The participation of endogenous melatonin in the normal sleep-wake cycle regulation has been inferred from the temporal relationships between melatonin cycle and the 24-hour cycle in sleep propensity, and particularly between the nocturnal melatonin onset and the nocturnal sleep gate (9-11). The typical 24-hour sleep propensity pattern reveals a midafternoon sleepiness peak followed by a forbidden zone for sleep, which is characterized by very low sleep propensity in the early evening hours and then followed by the nocturnal sleep gate.[14]

Serotonin is synthesized through 2-step process involving a tetrahydro-biopterin-dependent *hydroxylation* reaction (catalyzed by *tryptophan-5-monooxygenase*) and then a *decarboxylation* catalyzed by *aromatic L-amino acid decarboxylase*. The hydroxylase is normally not saturated and as a result, an increased uptake of tryptophan in the diet will lead to increased brain serotonin content.[15]

Serotonin is present at highest concentrations in platelets and in the gastrointestinal tract. Lesser amounts are found in the brain and the retina. Serotonin containing neurons have their cell bodies in the midline raphe nuclei of the brain stem and project to portions of the hypothalamus, the limbic system, the neocortex and the spinal cord. After release from serotonergic neurons, most of the released serotonin is recaptured by an active reuptake mechanism.

Melatonin is derived from serotonin within the pineal gland and the retina, where the necessary *N-acetyltransferase enzyme* is found. The pineal parenchymal cells secrete melatonin into the blood and cerebrospinal fluid. Synthesis and secretion of melatonin increases during the dark period of the day and is maintained at a low level during daylight hours. *This diurnal variation in melatonin synthesis is brought about by norepinephrine secreted by the postganglionic sympathetic nerves that innervate the pineal gland. The effects of norepinephrine are exerted through interaction with β-adrenergic receptors. This leads to increased levels of cAMP, which in turn activate the N-acetyltransferase required for melatonin synthesis.*

---

[14] http://www.nel.edu/23_3/NEL230302A02_Luboshitzky.htm
[15] http://web.indstate.edu/thcme/mwking/aminoacidderivatives.html

Melatonin synthesis

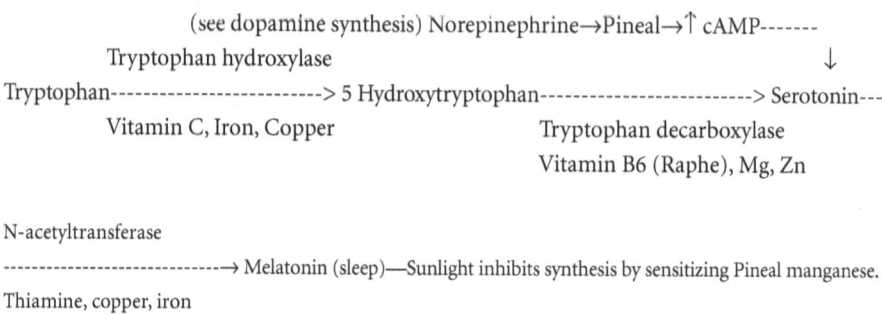

(see dopamine synthesis) Norepinephrine→Pineal→↑ cAMP------

Tryptophan hydroxylase   ↓

Tryptophan------------------------> 5 Hydroxytryptophan------------------------> Serotonin---

Vitamin C, Iron, Copper   Tryptophan decarboxylase

Vitamin B6 (Raphe), Mg, Zn

N-acetyltransferase

----------------------------→ Melatonin (sleep)—Sunlight inhibits synthesis by sensitizing Pineal manganese.

Thiamine, copper, iron

A person with bipolar disease will probably have lower amounts of phosphate ion. The result is a larger amount or different ratio of cAMP compared to ATP. The substance cAMP only possesses one phosphate compared to the three the ATP possesses. With higher levels of cAMP more melatonin would be synthesized producing drowsiness or sleep. A person with this disease would probably have difficulty falling aseep because of tryptophan hydroxlase deficiency, but once they fall asleep they be expected to sleep long and hard. I believe this is true and I have experienced this phenomenon.

I do not recommend taking copper without supervision. Copper can be very toxic. I only take 1 capsule each night at bedtime. My son and I tended to have **insomnia**. He hands trembled also. This is known as **essential tremor**. There are two types of copper. It is the oxidized green type of copper, not the red penny type we are used to seeing, which is active in the body. Absorption of copper is better if it is in the form of an organic salt, as opposed to highly ionized copper oxide. Copper oxide is the most prevalent type found in drug store vitamins. This form is not absorbed well.

I was aware that insufficient dopamine produced similar hand tremors in Parkinson patients. You know, the Michael J. Fox disease. I also learned of a disease called Wilson's. This disease produces hand tremors. Wilson's disease is a disease of copper metabolism. There is a decrease in serum copper and excess in overall copper due to copper being deposited at organ sites because of a failure of the copper to be released into bile for excretion.[16] I learned that copper was involved in two sequences in the production of

---

[16] http://digestive.niddk.nih.gov/ddiseases/pubs/wilson/index.htm

dopamine. The first is phenylalanine to tyrosine via a copper mediated enzyme called phenylalanine hydroxylase. Tyrosine is converted to L-Dopa with the help of vitamin C and the enzyme tyrosine hydroxylase. L-Dopa is converted to dopamine with the help of vitamin B6 and phosphate. The other pathway involved conversion of tyrosine to dopa via a copper enzyme called tyrosinase.[17] **Tyrosine hydroxylase** catalyzes the rate-limiting step in the biosynthesis of the catecholamines dopamine, norepinephrine, and epinephrine. Therefore, the regulation of tyrosine hydroxylase enzyme number and intrinsic enzyme activity represents the central means for controlling the synthesis of these important biogenic amines.[18]

Note the frequency with which the word *hydroxylase* comes up in this book. It is frequent and this leads me to believe that many of the hydroxylase enzymes are affected in this disease.

I did not know if this would work or not, but I decided to give it a try. I again went to the health food store and purchased absorbable copper. It is important to note that the type of copper is very important. It must be absorbable, the green type of copper and not the penny red we are so familiar. This green copper is better absorbed like most minerals if is in a neutral organic form. **He tried this and the tremors miraculously went away.**

Copper and manganese are primarily excreted via the bile. *As I would learn later, excessively reabsorbed chlorine causes down regulation of bile production.* This probably results in lower levels of these elements. Consequently, you see tremors from decreased dopamine production because of lower copper levels. You also see **increased bleeding times** caused by lower levels of manganese, which is involved with vitamin K, the clotting vitamin.

Beware that other diseases are associated with copper metabolism and they must be excluded before starting copper supplementation. These diseases include Wilson's disease and Menke's disease. These diseases are associated copper deposition in body organs. Copper supplements are should not be used in these conditions. [19]

As I investigated I found that copper is the cofactor needed for the conversion of tryptophan to melatonin. Most people recognize tryptophan from

---

[17] http://www.biochemj.org/bj/333/0685/3330685.pdf

[18] http://www.jneurochem.org/cgi/content/abstract/67/2/443

[19] Merck Manual, Fifteen Edition, page 947.

their yearly gorging of turkey at Thanksgiving and the nap that follows this feast. Melatonin is the substance necessary for the production of sleep. If a person's copper level is low, then inevitably their sleep will suffer. The vitamin thiamine plays a vital role in this process. It is thiamine that is converted to tryptophan. When the levels of thiamine and copper are appropriate the body will produce enough melatonin to induce sleep. In a normal person this level is reached at about 9:30 p.m. Since beginning this therapy, I get a very strong sleep urge at this time.

Sleep deprivation is a real problem with bipolar patients. In times of stress the body and mind's nutrient requirement is higher. If ingestion of necessary nutrients is insufficient and excretion is hyper-efficient, then the risks for metabolic failure in certain pathways are high. The excessive loss of copper results in the failure to induce sleep. Excessive sleep deprivation may evolve into psychosis. This may be because at a point the body begins producing a substance similar to LSD. Auditory and visual hallucinations may begin. It is important to note that copper comes in different forms. Some are absorbed from the gut and some are not. I have tried supplements found in the drug store that contained the non-absorbed form copper oxide. It was only after I tried the absorbable form that I achieved results. The organic copper forms are less ionized and, therefore, have better absorption characteristics. Note that copper is involved in all the body's oxidation reactions. Oxidation reactions are chemical reactions that involve oxygen.

The relationship between renal tubular acidosis (RTA) and copper metabolism has been investigated in a group of 18 patients with primary biliary cirrhosis. RTA, considered when unary PH remained above 5.4 after an oral load of ammonium chloride of 0.1 g/kg body wt, ws found in 6 patients (33%). Plasma copper concentration ((PCu) and urinary copper excretion (UCuV) were significantly higher in patients with RTA (PCu=182.2micrograms/dl, UCuV=536.8 micrograms/24 h) than in those without (PCu=134.2;UCuV=170.3). Plasma copper concentration and urinary copper excretion correlated with minimal urinary pH achieved after the ammonium chloride load. A higher degree of cholestasis was present in patients with RTA than in those without, and a linear correlation was observed between PCu and UCuV and serum bilirubin. It is concluded that the increased UCuV is related to the cholestasis in primary biliary cirrhosis and that the RTA might be caused by deposition of copper in the distal renal tubule.[20]

---

[20] http://www.ncbi.nlm.nih.gov/entrez

Copper is also important in calcium regulation. "Copper is the cofactor for the enzyme that does the cross-linking of collagen. In the laboratory if you create that copper deficiency they develop a bone lesion similar to osteoporosis."[21]

Copper deficiency may produce anemia or "iron poor blood." Copper deficiency causes low ceruloplasmin, which results in iron deficiency anaemia because of ferroxidase activity, is lost. Copper deficiency causes movement disorders and hypotonia resulting from disruption of dopamine synthesis due to disruption of dopamine beta-hydroxylase activity. Copper deficiency causes loss of lysyl oxidase, which impairs the cross linking of collagen, and elastin and this explains the impairment of vascular integrity and growth. Copper deficiency inhibits tyrosinase and hence melanin production is reduced. Copper deficiency may also cause defective myelin synthesis, impair glucose tolerance, and hypercholesterolaemia.[22]

Copper, also, helps in the formation of dopamine, the central nervous system neurotransmitter responsible for filtering incoming stimulus. We can go back to our electrical appliance analogy and derive that a telephone answering machine serves a similar purpose. Without enough dopamine the mind races unable to distinguish important stimuli from unimportant stimuli. For example, with "call-waiting" we can distinguish that important phone number to answer from annoying phone solicitors. When the level of dopamine is low the mind races to process all the stimuli. The mind becomes overwhelmed and the messages get confused. For the cooks, think of dopamine as a colander. You are rinsing your spaghetti noodles and normally the water passes over the spaghetti while the colander keeps the spaghetti. However, without dopamine the holes of the colander are too large and the spaghetti falls into the sink.

Fructose, the sweetener found in soft drinks, is a potent copper antagonist.[23] My son would drink a 6 pack of non-cola drinks containing the sweetener, high fructose corn syrup, after football practice in South Carolina. The South Carolina sun punished his body more than opposing players. Each day after practice I would pick him up and he would be drenched in sweat. I eventually realized that fructose had been shutting down his copper pathways. We originally stopped all fructose related drinks. We have now resumed use in small infrequent quantities

---

[21] http://www.orthopedictechreview.com/issues/julaug00/page30.htm

[22] http://www.gpnotebook.co.uk/cache/-502923221.htm

[23] www.thenutritionreporter.com/fructose_dangers.html

since his condition has improved dramatically. Orange juice, water, and diet colas have become the common drinks in our household. The one saving grace of cola drinks is that they contain phosphoric acid, which can supply needed phosphate to the body. I believe that the original maker of Coca Cola was on the right track in that he recognized the importance of bicarbonate and phosphate. I will point out the he too was a pharmacist.

Note that at least 8 mg of zinc is lost in sweat each day in an average athlete.[24] I estimate this amount is probably higher in athletes with bipolar disease. Without zinc, the body becomes acidic because carbonic anhydrase fails.

It is important for athletes to understand the physical limits that bipolar disease places on their bodies. This does not mean they should stop their athletic activity, but that it is more important to have an even better understanding of bipolar disease because of the extreme mineral losses and dehydration associated with this activity. Proper hydration is absolutely essential for the bipolar athlete.

Copper is also important in the performance of vitamin D and parathyroid hormone. *Vitamin D, parathyroid hormone and insulin are all related compound-sathlete*.[25] The copper connections lead me to vitamin D. This led me to parathyroid hormone, PT. Parathyroid hormone controls the absorption of calcium from the gut by its action on vitamin D. *Vitamin D selects calcium from the gut uniquely from the other available ions.* Once I found the parathyroid pathway, I reviewed the parathyroids actions. I found out this hormone also stimulates calcium reabsorption in the kidneys. This finding intrigued me. I had always considered bipolar disease to be a mental illness. I wondered, "Why was the parathyroid taking me to the kidneys?" I had always considered the kidneys to be an innocuous filter. I really didn't think there was much to it. Water in, water out…until you get old or the kidney quits functioning. I was ignorant.

As strange as it may sound there are considerable similarities between bipolar disease and menopausal symptoms. We are familiar with the emotional lability of women going through menopause. Those emotions of anger and depression are expressed in both diseases. In both conditions there is a loss of calcium and phosphate. If we conclude that these are similar conditions, then the explanation for copper loss may be explained.

---

[24] http://surgery.mc.duke.edu/nutrition/secure/trace_elements.html
[25] http://surgery.mc.duke.edu/nutrition/secure/trace_elements.html

"...Osteoporosis potentiates an acquired adult copper deficiency...Copper is the cofactor for the enzyme that does the cross-linking of collagen. In laboratory, if you create that copper deficiency, then bone lesions develop similar to osteoporosis.[26] Serum copper deficiency has been linked to essential tremor.[27] Therefore, **essential tremor** may be useful diagnosing bipolar disease. Copper deficiency ultimately will result in dopamine deficiency and the corresponding dopamine deficient mental symptoms. Remember, dopamine acts as a filter. Imagine dopamine as an usher taking tickets to the latest blockbuster movie. The usher takes a break and anyone who wants to see the movie enters the theater. Obviously, there would not be enough room for all the people and chaos would result. A similar situation exists when dopamine is insufficient.

Copper deficiency may cause seizures. Note that seizures may occur in psychotic patients. Anticonvulsants may increase serum levels of copper. [28] Anticonvulsants, as we shall learn, also decrease levels of vitamin D.

[26] http://www.orthopedictechreview.com/issues/julaug001/page30.htm.

[27] http://digestive.niddk.nih.gov/ddiseases/pubs/wilson/index.htm

[28] http://neuro-www.mgh.harvard.edu/forum/EpilepsyF/
11.22.973.29AMEpilepsyNutritio

CHAPTER 7

Mood

The moody blues, GABA deficiency

I had always been a very moody person. I remember one time a guy said, "No one really knows what you are going to be like, up or down." It hurt a little bit at the time, but he was right. I would have great days where I was smiling, telling jokes, and just enjoying life, which would be followed with a dour, mournful persona that simply "wore people out". It was easy to find friends when I was up, but when the melancholy hit they would run for the door. They distrusted me and I learned to distrust them. This behavior inevitably brings on isolation. Isolation is a tremendous weakness. There is tremendous wisdom in the expression "no man is an island". Society by its very definition demands integration. Integration into society enhances self-preservation. Therefore, I believe it is a primal instinct to be with others. These mood swings are more than just an innocuous affect. They can dissolve the bonds that tie the person to society and toss these unfortunate souls into the labyrinth of sub-culture.

I had performed an Internet search on "**mood.**" I found some interesting information concerning manganese. Manganese is an element of the earth. If inhaled it can cause toxicity. But, **ingested in small quantities (trace element) it acts as a catalyst in the conversion of alpha ketoglutamate to gamma amino butyric acid, also known as GABA. GABA is the substance that gives a person a feeling of well-being.** It is increased when small to moderate amounts of alcohol are consumed. So the laughing and smiling faces you see at parties is the result of GABA production. Years earlier, I had prescription eyeglasses called Photo Gray Extras that contained manganese. These eyeglasses would change color. They were normal in room light, but they would darken when exposed to sunlight. Scientists refer to this as photosensitivity. After connecting manganese to mood and manganese to sunlight I researched ultraviolet light. I found that the states lowest in UV were West Virginia and Vermont and the highest were California and Hawaii.[29] No wonder they are called "laid back Californians". I found that tea has high levels of manganese.[30] I fixed a breakfast of eggs and bacon and I made some "sun tea". I had learned that tea contains a high amount of manganese. The family had gathered outside on the deck in the summer sun and we drank tea. My son and a friend went for a walk at the park.

Startling was the effect on my son's eyes. His eyes had been very dilated for several months, even in bright sunshine. **A sign of agitation is the symptom dilated pupils.** That afternoon, however, his eyes were very normal. Eureka!

I had trouble repeating this experiment. I would learn later, it is <u>magnesium and acetylcholine</u> that controls eye dilation. Apparently, he received enough magnesium from an unidentified source. The acetylcholine is found in eggs. In my mind though it did not matter because his eyes, at least for this day, had normalized. I felt confident I would find the answer and I did.

In my research of the parathyroid I looked up hypoparathyroidism and hyperparathyroidism, low and high respectively. I found that in hyperparathyroidism the treatment was magnesium. I theorized that magnesium must play a more important role in mood than I had anticipated. I now wanted biochemical pathways that contained mineral cofactors. I found Roche Biochemical Pathways, an Internet site known as Expasy.

This is an extremely detailed Website with a multitude of metabolic reactions. My intuition was correct. I found that both magnesium and manganese play pivotal roles in catalyzing the production of GABA. My psychiatrist had mentioned years earlier that magnesium seemed to be promising for bipolar treatment. However, positive results had occurred only sporadically. This was probably because the most readily available product at the time was magnesium chloride. The trouble is that the chloride ion made the condition worse by creating apprehension and anxiety as well as encouraging acidosis.

Almost all of us have experienced GABA's effects if we have had an alcoholic drink. The pathway, as I see it, is that alcohol cleaves magnesium from its protein bound complex making more magnesium available for other reactions. This helps to produce more GABA and, therefore, "well being." As the party progresses, however, available magnesium is depleted and the levels of GABA

---

[29] http://www.nws.noaa.gov
[30] www.orst.edu/dept/lpi/infocenter/phytochemicals

decline. Since those magnesium stores have been depleted the partier awakens feeling worse for the wear so to speak.

Manganese acts as a catalytic co-factor for the vitamins pyridoxine, biotin, and pantothenic acid. Pyridoxine is especially important too in the production of serotonin, the up and Adam substance. Decarboxylation of glutamate produces GABA (*gamma*-aminobutryate).[31]

Zinc acts with pyridoxine to synthesize GABA (mood) in the brain. Riboflavin, cobalt, zinc, and manganese are all involved in the activation of pyridoxine.

---

[31] http://www.sbuniv.edu/~ggray.wh.bol/CHE3364/b1c25out.html

Weight loss, Attention Deficit, Dilated Eyes, Depression, and Exercise Intolerance

Why is a growing teenager losing weight? Glycolysis

Why was my growing teenage son losing weight? This was one of many questions I asked myself. I was familiar with glycolysis. Weight loss is expected during periods of extended glycolysis and gluconeogenesis. Glycolysis is a method of utilizing glucose when oxygen is unavailable. It is believed that control of glycolysis is primarily vested in the enzyme phosphofructokinase. Its activity is accelerated under conditions of tissue hypoxia. Accelerated glycolysis leads to overproduction of pyruvic acid, a strong acid.[32] Hypoxia is a medical term to describe insufficient levels of oxygen.

Once I made this association, up came the windows and in came the plants. I learned that English Ivy was a wonderful oxygen generator. My response was much like the character playing Sandra Bullock's mother, Gina Rowlands, in the movie Hope Floats. When Sandra is depressed and lying around in dark room her mother comes in draws the curtains and opens the window and tells

---

[32] Harrison's Principles of Internal Medicine, 10th Edition, pages 679, 680.

Sandra, "You are not going to hideout." So don't let your loved ones "hideout". Take them for a drive with the windows open. Let them breath the fresh air they were designed to breath. Go for a walk with them in the morning to let them soak up the sunshine their bodies crave. A very detailed explanation of glycolysis exists in Chapter 14, Phosphate.

Vitamin B6 functions as a co-enzyme for glycogen phosphorylase, an enzyme that catalyzes the release of glucose stores in muscle as glycogen. This process is known as glycolysis. Vitamin B6 is also used to generate glucose from amino acids. This process is known as gluconeogenesis. The failure to generate glucose through glucoenogenesis may be the reason for carbohydrate cravings in bipolar people.

Ketone bodies (acetoacetic acid, 3-hydroxybutyrate) are acids, which can cause a decrease in blood pH. (Ketone bodies have been implicated in causing mild depression in people losing weight). **These acids are also relative to beta-Oxidation Pathway hyperactivity.**[33] Ketone bodies are produced during periods of severe starvation. Hypoglycemia or low blood sugar is just such a period. Frequent sugar loads may produce frequent hypoglycemic reactions. Therefore, ketone bodies may accumulate to make you "stupid" or depressed.

"ATP produced by glycolysis is predominantly utilized for vesicular accumulation of Glu in the nerve ending. Synaptic vesicles are capable of accumulation Glu via activation of endogenous GADPH/2PGK."[34] This means that *when there is not enough glucose in the body more glutamate is accumulated.* Imagine you are in a boat in the ocean. It is calm and your boat sails over these normal sized waves with ease. This describes your glucose levels when you eat low glycemic foods. Imagine a tidal wave comes crashing down and your boat capsizes. You swim for your life. A high glucose load produces the same type of effect, hyperglycemic wave followed by hypoglycemic ebb. When multiple tidal waves occur frequently the results can be devastating. Sugar induced hypoglycemic waves, according to this article, are causing a significant rise in glutamate, which results in attention deficits. *Why are these foods allowed in our schools?*

To serve as additional buffers, the cell of the renal tubules generate ammonia (a neurotoxin) largely from the *hydrolysis of glutamine.*[35] This fact may serve as the "smoking gun" in the explanation of attention deficits.

The high levels of pyruvic acid are converted into glutamate. High levels of glutamate have been implicated in attention deficit disorder. This is probably

---

[33] http://www.sbuniv.edu/~ggray.wh.bol/CHE3364/b1c25out.html
[34] http://www.jbc.org/content/full/278/8/5929
[35] Harrison's Principles of Internal Medicine, 10th Edition, page 1605.

the result of increased neurotoxin ammonia produced from glutamate metabolism to glutamine. Glutamate is an amino acid that acts as an excitatory neurotransmitter. **Magnesium does inhibit the excitatory effect of glutamate.** "The excitatory amino acids glutamate (glu) and aspartate (asp) are thought to be the major excitatory transmitters. All of this explained why his grades were falling. So the first thing I did was open his window and I bought some houseplants to freshen the air. I encouraged him to go for walks.

Magnesium is necessary for acetylcholine to modulate attention. My son began to experience severe **attention deficits.** His grades plummeted. Note, too, that his eyes had become extremely dilated. This is a sign of agitation. It is also probably a sign of attention deficit. The vitamin pathway that was failing was pantothenic acid. Pantothenic acid and magnesium and/or manganese interact to produce acetylcholine.

His exercise tolerance had declined significantly as well. Magnesium and pantothenic acid is required for the energy producing reactions involving AMP, ADP, and ATP. The metallic co-enzyme for the vitamin Pantothenic acid appears to magnesium and manganese. Pantothenic acid is an essential component of co-enzyme A. Pantothenic acid provides the acyltransfer cofactor for many enzymatic reactions. Pantothenic acid is involved in the production of **acetylcholine, melatonin and heme.** (Acetylcholine is an important central excitatory neurotransmitter that monitors a person's attention; melatonin is involved with sleep; and heme is involved in blood formation. Pyridoxine is also involved in heme formation).

Acetylcholine stimulates ADH, antidiuretic hormone which prevents excessive urinary excretion, production in the SON, supra orbital nucleus of the eye. (As we have seen, magnesium and acetylcholine may correct dilated eyes). Pantothenic acid is involved with manganese in cholesterol production and steroid synthesis. A deficiency results in **"burning feet", decreased exercise tolerance,** decreased glycogen, and decreased myelin sheath. The derivative pantothenate has cholesterol-lowering effects. Food sources include: fish, tuna, chicken, egg, milk, bread, and yogurt. [36]

---

[36] Merck Manual, Fifteenth Edtion, 1987, page 939

Pantothenic acid is involved in energy metabolism and accepts phosphate ion from ATP, ADP, and AMP.

Selenium is a mineral involved in re-oxidation of glutathione. I have included selenium here because selenium deficiency is associated with neuronal death. It shares a close metabolic relationship with Vitamin E. In absence of selenium, lipid peroxides and free radicals may damage cell membranes. Acidosis potentiates oxidative neuronal death by multiple mechanisms. Acidosis has been found to potentiate markedly neuronal death induced by H202, peroxide, exposure. **Acidosis was found to reduce the activities of glutathione peroxidase (selenium) and glutathione S transferase by 50 to 60 percent...via direct inhibition of glutathione.** [37]

Sugar loading produces a "tidal wave" of glucose. This rapidly absorbed "tidal wave of glucose" is also metabolized extremely rapidly. This "tidal wave of glucose" plummets. The result is a condition known as hypoglycemia. This means the body is now "running on empty." The body reacts for survival by producing energy products, like glucose and others, from body stores of fat and protein. The survival methods utilized are known as glycolysis and gluconeogenesis. The hypoglycemia induced glycolysis increases glutamate production. Hypoglycemia will also strongly stimulate the urge to eat. Therefore, the dangerous cycle of "sugar high, sugar low" repeats again. The glutamate accumulates producing attention deficits. Consumption of fat or protein may prevent this hypoglycemic reaction because they are slowly absorbed and metabolized

---

[37] http://surgery.mc.duke.edu/nutrition/secure/trace_elements.html

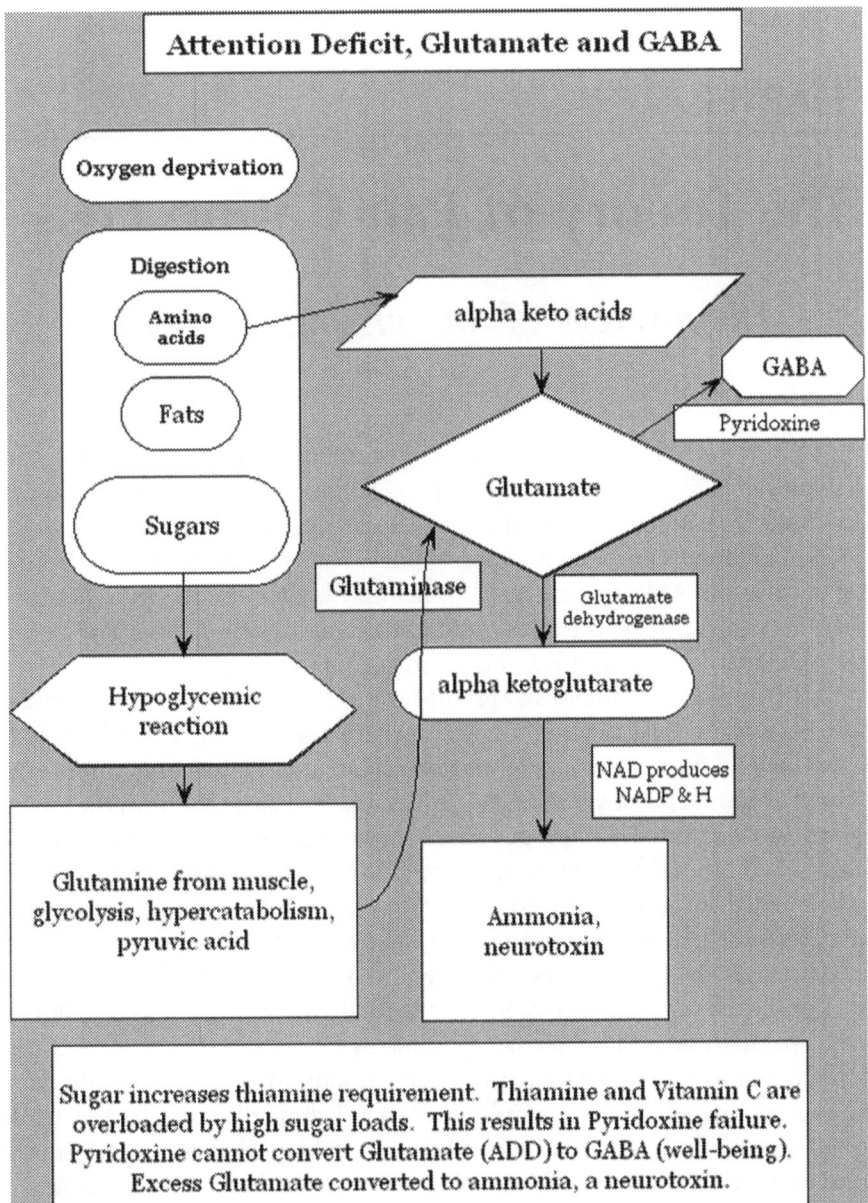

Attention Deficit, Glutamate and GABA

Oxygen deprivation

Digestion
- Amino acids
- Fats
- Sugars

alpha keto acids

GABA

Pyridoxine

Glutamate

Glutaminase

Glutamate dehydrogenase

Hypoglycemic reaction

alpha ketoglutarate

NAD produces NADP & H

Glutamine from muscle, glycolysis, hypercatabolism, pyruvic acid

Ammonia, neurotoxin

Sugar increases thiamine requirement. Thiamine and Vitamin C are overloaded by high sugar loads. This results in Pyridoxine failure. Pyridoxine cannot convert Glutamate (ADD) to GABA (well-being). Excess Glutamate converted to ammonia, a neurotoxin.

CHAPTER 9

The Theory of Pan-Cation Loss

The mystery of the missing elements

I had purchased an ugly yellow piece of poster board to put my findings in some kind of logical order. I would write each discovery onto the board in the place under a main topic like sleep. Once I accumulated enough items under a topic I placed them in sequential order. I now had a simple schematic beginning in darkness. As I said before, I began with the very basics. This schematic ran to daylight. It then converged with glutamate to form GABA and so on. One night after looking at this I noticed something unusual.

What I found was minerals kept appearing in key points in the pathway. There they were zinc, magnesium, manganese and copper. I hypothesized, **"Something is causing the loss of all these elements."** I knew only three ways this could occur (1) decreased intake, (2) decreased absorption from the gut or (3) increased excretion. I knew decreased intake did not fit because I ate voraciously. I did not feel that decreased absorption from the gut fit because normally in malabsorption syndromes diarrhea plays a pivotal role. I would later learn of a probable malabsorption pathway from a down-regulated bile system. Although I had diarrhea occasionally it was not on a daily basis plus I had not experienced any weight loss. So I looked hard at excretion. I asked, "What was the parathyroid and kidney trying to tell me?"

In the meantime, my regimen now included sodium bicarbonate, zinc, copper, and manganese. My son would not take all these pills so I had to work around this by finding foods he liked that were high in these ingredients. I found that food in cashews, which are high in zinc, copper and manganese.

The mineral manganese is photosensitive. That means it responds to light. I used to have eyeglasses that contained this mineral. The lenses would darken when exposed to light and become clear when light was less available. Manganese is also found in the pineal gland close to the retina.

I believe that in darkness manganese in the pineal gland becomes less active. This result allows synthesis of melatonin to proceed. The consequence is sleep. As sleep progresses to around 4 a.m. cortisol is secreted. Cortisol is a steroid that is produced by the adrenal gland. Cortisol secretion, I expect, causes a slight increase in circulating minerals, which is probably from cortisol acting on the bone or gall bladder. Manganese is the mineral, I believe, that is most active here. The increase in manganese makes the pineal more sensitive to light. The result of the sun rising above the horizon is awakening. This is all theory of course.

I continued my research by studying Roche Biochemical Pathways. I found that magnesium was required for GABA synthesis, which would "calm the savage beast." I found food sources such as avacado and Brazil nuts, but he did not desire them so I went to the health food store and I was shown a product called Natural Calm. This is a powder form of magnesium citrate. I began putting it in orange juice and it has a tarty taste. He liked it at first. Soon the anger went away, but the pupils of his eyes were still large. I reviewed other articles and I found that **acetylcholine and magnesium regulate pupil size. Acetylcholine is found in eggs.** So I cooked breakfast and I gave him his orange juice. Ouila, his eyes normalized. Now real progress was happening.

CHAPTER 10

The Kidneys

Mineral gatekeeper

The kidneys, that mean two, are the filter system for the fluid in the body. The kidney performs a variety of functions including picking out which mineral to keep and which to throw away. These functions are referred to as reabsorption and excretion. The kidney is also involved in the formation of blood. It is also involved in the activation of vitamin D to regulate calcium and phosphate metabolism. If one kidney is bad this can throw everything out of whack. The body has a host of ways to compensate for this malfunction, but they can come with adverse effects. If one kidney is only slightly injured while the other is intact this can produce a small "leak" of minerals. In other words, this kidney is throwing stuff away while the healthy kidney tries to adjust. The parathyroid gland makes many of these adjustments. The parathroid gland is responsible for calcium and phosphate regulation. I believe this is what occurs in bipolar illness.

I pondered, "The kidneys, the kidneys?" I began reviewing my Harrison's Principles of Internal Medicine for clues. After reviewing many sections on the kidney I stumbled across one disease that made sense, distal Renal Tubular Acidosis. I think we are all familiar with the term acid. Acidosis is a term used to describe a condition where too many hydrogen atoms in an ionized state exist in the body. Harrison's Principles of Internal Medicine describes this disease as, "group of disorders where renal excretion is reduced out of proportion to any reduction of glomerular filtration rate that may be present. Metabolic acidosis results, but in contrast to renal failure, the anions that accompany surplus hydrogen ions in the blood, such as sulfate and phosphate, are excreted normally and are unavailable to balance any fall in serum bicarbonate that occurs. Therefore, the kidneys reabsorb chloride in unusually large amounts, and serum chloride rises to preserve electroneutrality n the extracellular fluid. The result is hyperchloremic acidosis, and the unmeasured anion gap is normal. There is general agreement that four types of RTA exist. Types 1 and 2 are often hereditary. Type 3 is a rare mixture of types 1 and 2. Type 4 is acquired…" Treatment includes: "Sodium bicarbonate tablets (10 grains=7.2 meq base) and Shohl's solution (1m eq base per milliliter, as Na and K citrate)."

The term hyperchloremic is an adjective used to describe the type of condition where too much chloride ion exists in the body. Hyper is a medical prefix used to express "too much". Hypo is a medical prefix used to express "too low." So we see that this person has too much chlorine floating around in their body.

I had not used bicarbonate during my lifetime because when I was a child I had heard of a gentleman who died of a heart attack after using bicarbonate of soda. I never used this product because of that fact. I had a headache one day at work and the only medicine we had in our little medicine cabinet was Alka Seltzer. I decided to give it a try. This medicine is a combination of bicarbonate and acetaminophen. I recall the tremendous cooling feeling I had from this medicine.

This made sense to me. The treatment for this disease included sodium bicarbonate and also potassium citrate. Potassium citrate? Isn't that in orange juice? Yes. So my regimen now included orange juice fortified with magnesium powder from the health food store, sodium bicarbonate, and cashews. I was doing better and my son was responding too. My son was happy and now enjoying activities he hadn't done in months and months, basically before puberty. He was going out with friends skateboarding. Interest in activities that had diminished reemerged.

Of all the types of kidney disorders I have reviewed this type appears to explain what is happening the best. This condition is called Rate-Limited Secretory distal Renal Tubular Acidosis.

This condition appears to be RATE-LIMITED SECRETORY RTA!!!

Secretory distal RTA will be associated with hypokalaemia (or sometimes, normokalaemia), and respond well to administration of alkali (e.g. Shohl's solution). Note that with classical type I RTA (gradient-limited secretory distal RTA) the urine pH will tend to be over 5.5, while with rate-limited secretory distal RTA, pH is often below 5.5. Be cautious in using urinary pH—urea-splitting organisms present in urine might raise pH, and any cause of volume or potassium depletion will also raise it remarkably).

One problem that can be confused with rate-limited secretory distal RTA is defective NH3 production. Giving bicarbonate and checking the urinary PCO2 can distinguish these. If there is a distal defect in hydrogen ion secretion, the urine PCO2 minus the blood PCO2 will be abnormally low (under 3.3kPA). Normally, alkalinization of the urine to a pH of over 7.0 by NaHCO3 administration results in bicarbonaturia, and this bicarbonate binds distally secreted hydrogen ions to form H_2CO_3. The H_2CO_3 in turn breaks down to form CO_2 and H_2O, resulting in a urinary PCO_2 of over 3.3kPa.

Amphotericin B toxicity may resemble gradient-limited secretory distal RTA, but here again, urine PCO_2—blood PCO_2 will be normal, in contrast to the low value found in gradient-limited secretory distal RTA.

If you are still unsure about the presence or absence of distal RTA, ammonium chloride loading has been used to distinguish between distal RTA (where urine pH fails to drop below 5.5) on the one hand, and proximal or type IV RTA on the other (where the pH drops). In rate-limited distal RTA, the pH should also drop.[38]

---

[38] http://www.anaesthetist.com/icu/elec/nagacid/htm

CHAPTER 11

The Blood Test and Cravings

Confirming proof of ion deficiency

I went to my regular doctor to have blood work performed. All of my blood work came back in normal limits. He told me before he had the nurse take my blood that everything would be normal except the glucose because I had just had breakfast. He was right. I noted something unusual, however. I had high normal sodium levels, but the levels for every other mineral were low normal. I also had low normal protein levels. I had low normal alkaline phosphatase and eosinophils levels. I recalled that in previous years my potassium and iron levels were low. This was confirming my hypothesis. If you have the minimum of everything the rate of metabolic reactions will be slowed dramatically.

An *analogy* would be that three men are building a car from scratch. They can get it finished, but it would reasonably take several months. However, if you have a factory full of men the time necessary to build the same car is probably less than a week. Also, the body up-regulates and down-regulates certain metabolic pathways to give the person the ability to function. An example of this would be the lower levels of protein aid in function by freeing protein-bound minerals. These free mineral ions would be available to catalyze reactions. Succinctly, less protein means less ability for protein mineral reaction. In the above car analogy, up-regulation and down-regulation can be looked at as providing or taking away tools. Tools cost a lot of money. Certainly, if those three men had tools that made them more efficient, then that time frame comparison could change radically. The body can improve biochemical synthesis by making the reactions more efficient in some pathways, but usually this is at the expense of another pathway.

I noticed a high normal sodium level and low normal levels on other cations in my blood work. I was not consuming high amounts of sodium. I asked, "Why were my sodium levels high?" <u>Sodium can be actively reabsorbed in the renal tubule and in the collecting via aldosterone.</u> Aldosterone is the principal mineralocorticoid hormone in the human body. It causes sodium and water retention in the distal tubule of the kidney and increased excretion of potassium. Since my blood pressure is normal I suspect it is not in the collecting duct but in the proximal portion of the renal tubule and possibly because its ionic partner, chloride, level is high.

After researching iron and anemia I read that kidney was responsible for red blood cell production.

Table 1

Tests ordered: CBC with Diff; Comprehensive Metabolic Panel; TSH; Iron

Result Name
CBC with Diff

test	result	limits	result/cause
WBC	5.50	4.0-10.5k/ul	**low normal (zinc)**
RBC	4.89	4.22-5.81 mil/ul	**low normal (iron, copper)**
Hemoglobin	14.30	13.0-17.0 g/dl	**low normal (zinc)**
MCV	43.40	39.0-52.0%	
MCHC	88.80	78.0-100.0 fl	
RDW	12.70	11.5-14.6%	
Platelet Count	198.0	150-400 k/ul	**low normal**
Granulocyte %	54	43-77%	
Absolute Gran	3.0	1.4-7.7 k/ul	
Lymph	34	12-46%	
Absolute Lymph	1.9	0.7-3.3 k/ul	
Mono %	9	3-11	**high normal (extrarenal D3)**
Absolute Mono	0.5	0.2-0.7 k/ul	
Eos	2	0-5%	
Absolute Eos	0.1	0.0-0.6 k/ul	**low normal(stress, cortisol)**
Baso%	1	0-1%	
Absolute Baso	0.0	0.0-0.1k/ul	

Comprehensive Metabolic Panel

Sodium	142	135-145 mEq/l	**high normal***
Potassium**	4.1	3.5-5.5 mE/l	**low normal**
Chloride*	105	96-112 mEq/l	normal

CO2*	27	19-32 mEq/l	normal
glucose*	113 h	70-110 mg/dl	high
BUN	15	6-23 mg/dl	normal
Creatinine**	1.1	0.5-1.7 mg/dl	normal
Bilirubin, Total	0.3	0.3-1.2 mg/dl	**low normal (iron deficiency anemia)**
Alkaline Phosphatase	43	39-117 u/l	**low normal(zinc deficiency)**
AST/SGOT#	12	0-37 u/l	**low normal**
ALT/SGPT#	15	0-40 u/l	**low normal**
Total Protein	6.9	6.0-8.3 g/dl	**low normal (Mg needed to synthesize protein)**
Albumin	4.4	3.5-5.2 g/dl	normal
Calcium	9.5	8.4-10.5 mg/dl	normal
TSH	2.347	.350-5.50uIu/ml	normal

...Test methodology is 3rd generation TSH...

Iron**&	94	42-165 ug/dl	**low normal**

*"Hyperaldosteronism promotes metabolic acidosis"[39]

* probably normalized from treatment with potassium citrate and sodium bicarbonate at time of test or corrected via respiration.

*test taken after breakfast

---

[39] Harrson's Principles of Internal Medicine, 10th Edition, page 228.

#these items have been abnormally low in previous test times

SGOT,SGPT are aminotransferases. SGPT is involved in alpha ketoglutarate metabolism.

&Iron or copper and vitamin C are necessary for hydroxylase production.

If you determine the mid-point in the normal limits field you will notice that all of my cations, except sodium, are low. You will also see that sodium is in the high normal range. You will see protein is in the low normal range as well as bilirubin, alkaline phosphatase, and absolute Eos (eosinophils). Platelets, WBC (white blood cells), and RBC (red blood cells) were also affected. I was surprised that chloride and CO_2 were both normal. I can only attribute that to the sodium bicarbonate supplement working or increased respiration correcting CO_2. Perhaps, by limiting table salt, sodium chloride, I decreased the availability of chloride ion. This test did not check for bicarbonate ion concentrations. I later found that respiration alkalosis or hyperventilation does occur during this process.

Many of these ions like calcium and magnesium are protein bound. Protein in bipolar patients tends to be on the low side, therefore, the real levels of an ion like calcium is much worse than the blood work reading. This condition increases higher levels of circulating minerals because most of the minerals are protein bound and, therefore, unavailable for use. **People with low protein levels but with normal levels of minerals on blood tests may still have insufficient levels of minerals.** (Tryptophan, the sleep adjunct, is also protein bound).

"In conclusion, the results of the present study demonstrate that the loss of weak acid secondary to hypoproteinemia is compensated for by an increase in chloride ion."[40] Decreased levels of protein, therefore, would make the metabolic acidosis even worse.

Over the years my blood tests stated abnormally low potassium levels and low iron levels, and abnormally high creatinine levels. This high creatinine level occurred while I was taking lithium carbonate. A high creatinine level may presage kidney damage.

---

[40] http://jap.physiology.org/cgi/content/full/84/5/1740

Iron deficiency produces anemia. The primary symptom of anemia is tiredness. Anemia is a disease caused by decreased levels of oxygen carrying red blood cells. Iron deficiency also produces sleep disturbances and restless leg syndrome.

The low potassium levels were detected while I was in the hospital getting treated for psychosis. I remember drinking orange juice at breakfast. Orange juice tasted like the best thing I had ever drank. This brings me to a discussion about cravings.

In most instances craving is a good thing. We have all experienced cravings. Craving causes the body to consume quantities of a substance that it needs to continue proper metabolism. We have all heard humorous stories of Monica Lewinsky consuming huge quantities of ice cream during her stressful ordeal. This may be a normal response to stress. Stress, as you will see, causes phosphate loss. This, I believe, produces a decrease in the level of glucose 6-phosphate. The body requires both ingredients. When one is deficient, like phosphate, the body continues to ask for all the ingredients. In this case, glucose and phosphate are requested. The result in Monica's case is excess glucose, which is stored as fat.

It is important to identify your cravings and discuss them with your doctor. Once enough of the needed substance has been ingested then the craving simply goes away. *A continued craving even after ample quantities have been ingested needs to be investigated.* I have noticed since beginning supplementation that my diet is more regulated. I have lost about 10 pounds without trying. This makes me theorize that overeating may be a response to a nutritional deficiency. In Monica's case, this deficiency was caused by stress. I expect that the American diet is low in many of the ions we have discussed. We compensate by eating. The trouble is these are low nutrient foods. The ratio of nutrient to carbohydrate intake is too low. The result is excess carbohydrate intake which is stored as fat.

CHAPTER 12

Proof of Ion Depletion

Where did they go? KIDNEY and BILE

I have not found one single source describing the loss of ions with metabolic acidosis. I had to research this section ion by ion. I believe, however, that in the interstitial cells of the kidney where water is split to produce the positive hydrogen ion and the negative hydroxide ion that carbonic anhydrase fails to convert carbon dioxide to bicarbonate. The result is excessive hydrogen ion which gets reabsorbed via the active Na/K pump. This would produce metabolic acidosis. The interstitium becomes negatively charged because of excess hydroxide ions. The now overly active Na/K pump pours in excessive amounts of positive potassium, which interacts with the negative hydroxide ion. This compound which is basic is then excreted probably passively which results in urine that is substantially less acidic than a normal persons. Therefore, urinary tract complications may occur. Since this condition produces a negatively charged interstitium, the positively charged ions in the cell may pass into the interstitium resulting in trace element losses. The deficits produced by this result in vitamin pathway failures since most of these vitamins depend on these elements as cofactors. **Thiamine and pyridoxine are both profoundly affected because they depend on cofactors and they are phosphate salts as well.** Since this condition results in a phosphate deficiency, then the activity of these vitamins would be severely diminished. The physical and mental symptoms of bipolar disease establish this.

Calcium
The acidic condition (metabolic acidosis) causes calcium to be dissolved from the bones. The calcium accumulates in the bloodstream and excess serum calcium is excreted by the kidneys causing a total body loss of calcium

and resulting in osteomalacia or rickets.[41] If an acidic condition causes calcium to be dissolved from the bones, then other ions in the bone would be dissolved as well, especially magnesium.

The effect that lithium exhibits may be from decreasing urinary excretion of calcium.[42] Lithium also causes a tremor. This tremor may be related to copper interference.

A study involving calcium excretion and exercise came to this result. In conclusion, our study demonstrated that *1)* strenuous exercise increased urinary calcium excretion by decreasing renal calcium reabsorption, *2)* urinary calcium excretion increased independent of osteoclast activation, and *3)* the mechanism resulting in post exercise hypercalciuria might simply involve non-cell-mediated physicochemical bone dissolution.

Two possible mechanisms could be responsible for the bone dissolution by exercise-induced lactic acidosis. One possibility is the cell-mediated osteoclastic bone resorption. If it were responsible for the change in urinary calcium excretion, one would expect a rise in urinary deoxypyridinoline as a marker of bone resorption. In contrast, there was a significant decrease in urinary deoxypyridinoline excretion when urinary calcium excretion significantly increased. It is, therefore, more likely that the mechanism resulting in postexercise hypercalciuria might simply involve non-cell-mediated physiochemical bone dissolution, which is the dissolution of a fraction of the crystalline calcium hydroxyapatite compartment, independent of osteoclast activation. Short-term acidosis as such observed in this study may induce non-cell-mediated physiochemical bone dissolution.

An alternative source might be via enhanced absorption of calcium from the gut. Our study was not designed to assess the effects of exercise-induced lactic acidosis on calcium absorption from the gut; however, this possibility would appear unlikely in view of the fact that most authors failed to detect an increase of intestinal calcium absorption in complete metabolic studies in acute and chronic metabolic acidosis.[43]

---

41 http://www.nlm.nih.gov/medline plus/ency/article/000493.html

42 http://jcem.endojournals.org/cgi/content/abstract/68/3/654

43 http://jap.physiology.org/cgi/content/full/83/4/1159

Caffeine intake also should be limited because caffeine will increase urinary calcium excretion. The ingestion of 34 ounces of caffeine will cause a loss of 1.6 mmol of total calcium, contributing to both hypercalciuria and osteoporosis[44]

Potassium
Type 1 Renal Tubular Acidosis causes retention of acid and is also associated with mild loss of potassium in the urine.[45]

Bicarbonate
Distal renal tubular acidosis (Type 1 RTA) is a disorder caused by a defect in the secretion of hydrogen ions in the distal renal tubule (the late portion of the kidney tubule). This causes a reduction in the reabsorption of bicarbonate into the bloodstream.[46]

Magnesium
Primary renal disorders cause hypomagnesaemia by decreased tubular reabsorption of magnesium by the damaged kidneys. This occurs in the diuretic phase of acute tubular necrosis, post obstructive diuresis, renal tubular acidosis.[47]

(Note that the active Na/K pump would be a magnesium driven ATP pump. The over activity of this pump would probably result in excess magnesium availability in the interstitium with resulting magnesium excretion).

Manganese
Manganese is excreted via the bile. (Possibly not affected, but increased bleeding times probably from vitamin K failure provides a correlation that suggests manganese loss).[48]

Copper
Urinary copper excretion was significantly higher in patients with RTA.[49] Primary excretion occurs via bile.

---

[44] http://author.emedicine.com/MED/topic1069.htm

[45] http://www.nlm.nih.gov/medlineplus/ency/article/000493.html

[46] http://www.nlm.nih.gov/medlineplus/ency/article/000493.htm

[47] http://www.barttersite.com/hypomagnesemia.htm

[48] http://lpi.oregonstate.edu/infocenter/minerals/manganese/index.html

[49] http://www.ncbI.nlm.nih.gov/entrez/

Zinc

Zinc is excreted in the urine in higher quantities during stress.[50] Central to maintenance of zinc homeostasis, however, is the gastrointestinal system, especially the small intestine, liver and pancreas.[51]

Chromium

Chromium is excreted in the urine. Chromium gives the urine an orange color. If excessive chromium is being excreted then that color will be deeper. This may be evidence of disease condition.[52]

Iron

Iron is excreted in the urine.[53]

Molybdenum

Molybdenum is excreted via the bile. Molybdenum is involved with xanthine oxidase, uric acid, and riboflavin.

Cobalt

Cobalt is excreted principally in the urine and also in the feces.[54]

Superoxide dismutases

Superoxide dismutases are compounds that prevent oxidative injury. These compounds contain the elements copper, zinc, manganese, and iron. All of these ions appear to be affected by RTA. Hydroxide ion has been linked to oxidative injury. [55] Note that all of these elements are involved in the sleep-wake cycle. In progressive bipolar disease these elements are depleted probably by urinary excretion.

Carbonic Anhydrase, Zinc

Carbonic anhydrases are enzymes containing zinc that convert water and carbon dioxide to hydrogen ion and **bicarbonate**. A deficiency of zinc results in **carbonic anhydrase inhibition.** Symptoms of carbonic anhydrase inhibition

---

[50] http://surgery.mc.duke.edu/nutrition/secure/trace_elements.html

[51] http://www.nutrition.org/cgi/content/full/130/5/1374S

[52] http://surgery.mc.duke.edu/nutrition/secure/trace_elements.html

[53] http://surgery.mc.duke.edu/nutrition/secure/trace_elements.html

[54] http://archive.food.gov.uk/committees/evm/papers/evm7.pdf

[55] http://ehpnet1.niehs.nih.gov/members/1994/Supl-10/farber-full.html

include: diarrhea, increased urinary frequency, loss of appetite, metallic taste, lump in throat, increased eye sensitivity to sunlight, loss of taste and smell, nervousness and irritability. Also, diabetes, gout, emphysema, kidney stones, low potassium, under active adrenal glands, and liver disease are conditions associated with carbonic anhydrase inhibition.[56] **Carbonic anhydrase failure is associated with deficient 1,25 dihydroxy vitamin D3.**

---

[56] http://www.nlm.nih.gov/medlineplus/druginfo/uspdi/202114.html

Table 2

VITAMIN	COFACTOR	ACTIONS & EFFECT
Thiamine, B1*	Magnesium	decarboxylates alpha keto acids GABA conversion (mood)
Thiamine, B1*	Copper	dopamine formation dopamine formation (tremors)
Thiamine, B1*	Copper Iron	converts tryptophan to melatonin transferase, Melatonin (sleep)
Niacin	Iron Magnesium	NAD coenzyme 1, NADP coenzyme 2 cell metabolism and redox reactions
Pyridoxine, B6*	Magnesium Zinc Copper*** Magnesium Zinc, Cobalt, Manganese	converts tryptophan to serotonin (awakening & mood) dopamine, NE, GABA production dehydrogenase**, mood & stress
Folic Acid	Zinc	synthesizes SAM SAM(mood)
Cyanocobalamin	Cobalt	+ B6 to decrease homocysteine stress tolerance
Biotin	Magnesium Manganese	carboxylates prevents depression and lethargy
Pantothenic Acid	Magnesium Manganese	acyltransfer cofactor acetylcholine>ADH production, melatonin (sleep), heme(blood), with ATP, ADP, &AMP

VITAMIN	COFACTOR	ACTIONS & EFFECT
Vitamin C	Copper Iron	redox, metabolizes phenyalanine, collagen formation, norepinephrine synthesis
Riboflavin	Copper	oxidative phosphorylation enhances Pyridoxine

** tyrosine hydroxylase
* denotes phosphate compounds
***pyridoxine is antagonized by penicillamine, a copper level reducer used in Wilson's disease.

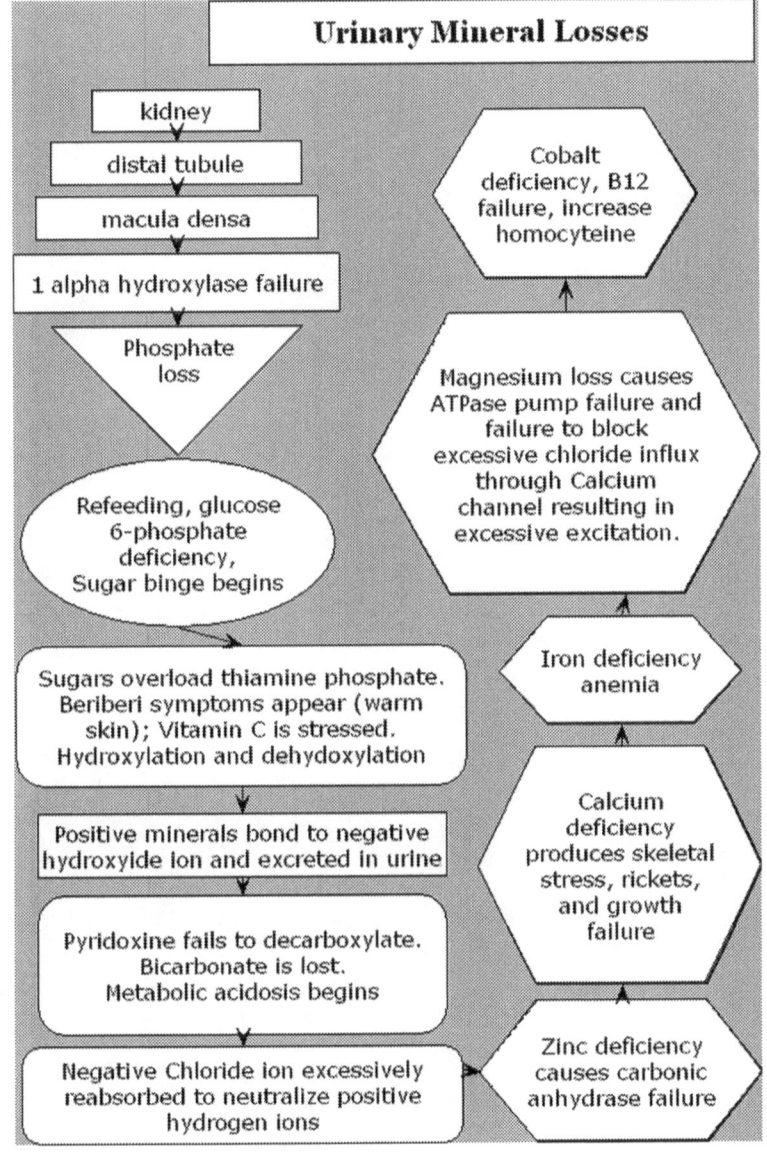

Urinary Mineral Losses

kidney

distal tubule

macula densa

1 alpha hydroxylase failure

Phosphate loss

Refeeding, glucose 6-phosphate deficiency, Sugar binge begins

Sugars overload thiamine phosphate. Beriberi symptoms appear (warm skin); Vitamin C is stressed. Hydroxylation and dehydoxylation

Positive minerals bond to negative hydroxyide ion and excreted in urine

Pyridoxine fails to decarboxylate. Bicarbonate is lost. Metabolic acidosis begins

Negative Chloride ion excessively reabsorbed to neutralize positive hydrogen ions

Cobalt deficiency, B12 failure, increase homocyteine

Magnesium loss causes ATPase pump failure and failure to block excessive chloride influx through Calcium channel resulting in excessive excitation.

Iron deficiency anemia

Calcium deficiency produces skeletal stress, rickets, and growth failure

Zinc deficiency causes carbonic anhydrase failure

SECTION 2

SYMPTOMS

CHAPTER 13

Colic, Sunken Chest, Scoliosis, Knock-kneed, Bow-legged and Bald-headed Babies

"You are such a big baby!" Calcium and Rickets

I was two weeks late at birth and I weighed ten pounds at birth. At six months I weighed 25 pounds. I also was a colicky baby. I believe that this disease creates *unbridled cravings* especially for calcium. My father would purchase 10 gallons of milk every Saturday for my two brothers, my sister, and myself. I was far and away the biggest *milk consumer* of the family. The weight gain is a result of the body being unable to satisfy the need for calcium and the calories that come with the calcium in milk lead to weight gain.

I had colic and my son had colic. My son was an extremely colicky baby. My wife had great difficulty pacifying him during the day. I would frequently come home from work and rock him until 3 in the morning. I believe this may be the reason the expression "You are such a big baby" was coined.

I had many *dental caries* as a child probably due to low calcium levels, *dry mouth*, and sweet cravings. I developed an *overbite*. My father, God rest his soul, spent a good portion of his life earnings in my mouth. I developed a *sunken chest*. I believe that both factors are related to this form of rickets. I believe that when the body does not have enough calcium to support certain skeletal structures it develops a more efficient way to make that structure which results in abnormality.

I believe *cravings* identify "ingredients" the body needs. The problem is that they usually come with calories. If the body cannot burn those calories weight gain occurs, therefore, the "fat baby". I have noticed since starting this therapy a very slow steady weight loss of about 10 pounds. This differs from weight loss via glycolysis because the weight lost is over a substantial period of time and apparently caused by a slight decrease in appetite. I do not eat the big bowel of ice cream anymore. A small one is just fine. *My cravings are substantially reduced.*

My blood pressure has always been about 133 over 72. The systolic pressure of 133 have not been of major concern, but since I have been on this therapy my systolic blood pressure has declined to 120. That means there is less aortic pressure…a good thing. *My systolic blood pressure has normalized.*

My *voice* used to be tired and raspy at times. It is now deep and resonant. This was, I believe, due to calcium loading readjusting my parathyroid hormone levels. *My voice is not raspy any longer.*

I have on a regular basis *right eye pain.* I believed this was because my eyes were tired. I mentioned this to my doctor one day and he said it is a form of migraine. I have learned to use this pain as a gauge of high PTH levels. When the pain occurs I realize it is time to calcium load. *I have reduced frequency and severity of right eye pain.*

I grew to be rather tall, but I believe *growth may be affected* in people with this disease. The skeleton can compensate for a lack of calcium, I believe, in two ways. The first way is to allow growth to progress normally and create more efficient development structures. These are usually defects like scoliosis, sunken chest, dental abnormalities, knock-knees, or bowed-legs. The second way is that if calcium levels fall to decrease the size of the skeleton. Therefore, there is a decreased need for calcium. In the latter case, you see short people. Randy Newman's song about short people is probably the result of him coming into contact with some short bipolar people. The interaction of a normal pituitary, a gland responsible for growth, with a parathyroid gland with widely varying rates of excretion may result in some unusual growth patterns.

In families with a prior history of the disease, the **absence of scalp hair in newborns** provides initial diagnostic evidence for HVDRR[57] (HVDRR stands for 1,25 dihydroxyvitamin D resistant rickets). My Mother said that I had plenty of hair when I was born, but it all fell out shortly after birth. My boys were bald when they were born. My grandson, on the other hand, had so much dark black hair when he was born his nickname was Elvis. I believe this symptom and colic can be valuable diagnostic tools, which can be used for identifying children with bipolar disease in early development. If pediatricians can identify children early in development then potential brain damage could be minimized. Imagine a society where an additional 1 or 2 percent of the population, many our best and brightest, is performing at their best.

---

[57] http://edrv.endojournals.org/cgi/content/full/20/2/156

CHAPTER **14**

Tired, Cold Intolerance, Lazy Eye, Sweet tooth, High Volume Urination, Thirst, Raspy Voice, Glycolysis and Glucose 6-Phosphate Deficiency

Phosphate, the energy ion

Imagine a cold night, you want to feel warm. You strike a match to create fire. The ingredient that started the match is phosphorus. This is also the same ingredient needed to give energy for life.

I developed *amblyopia* or lazy eye perhaps as a result of low phosphate. I believe that with the decreased energy levels associated with phosphate deficiency cold intolerance is expected. In order to tolerate cold you need a lot of energy. A person with bipolar disease will probably avoid outdoor related activities where cold tolerance is a necessity.

I was a good athlete but my performance would decline significantly in the 4th quarter of a basketball game or in the last set of a tennis match. I once scored 28 points in a half of basketball against former college players in a men's league game. Another time I beat the junior New Zealand champion in tennis. His brother was a circuit professional who took Jimmy Connors to three sets. So there were times I could perform at a very high athletic level. Usually, however, I would "disappear" late into a game or match. Many times my losses to much less talented players would leave me frustrated and shaking my head. I believe many of these losses were associated with loss of energy, again phosphate, and high stress sensitivity.

In college we had an experiment where we needed urine. I was given a 500ml glass beaker and I filled it up completely. My classmates' volume was maybe 100ml. This illustrates a deficiency in antidiuretic hormone. This also may explain the crude expression "pissing away your life" or at least your energy. Because of the potent phosphaturic nature of PTH combined with low ADH the result is a high volume of phosphate urine. *I have noticed since starting calcium loading that the quantity and frequency of urination has declined substantially.* I used to go to a restaurant and drink four or five large glasses of tea. Since I started this program I drink normal quantities, one or two glasses. *My thirst has normalized.*

My *voice* used to be tired and raspy at times. It is now deep and resonant. This was, I believe, due to Calcium loading readjusting my parathyroid hormone levels. *My voice is not raspy any longer.*

Note that phosphate is actively reabsorbed via sodium pump in the upper portion of the descending limb. This pump is sensitive to parathyroid hormone. In an attempt to maintain calcium levels the body requests intake of more calcium. The major source for calcium nutrition is obtained by drinking milk. Everyone is probably saying, "Well, this a good thing." There is a problem there however. Milk is now fortified with vitamin D. A person with bipolar disease who consumes extremely large quantities of milk will from time to time experience vitamin D toxicity. This toxicity produces its own set of problems.

Identifying the role of genetics in bipolar disease has proven difficult. Several reports by Mendlewicz and colleagues [146] produced sizable lod scores *linking bipolar disorder with color blindness and G6PD deficiency.*[58] This evidence helps to substantiate my theory because glucose 6 phosphate deficiency or G6PD is a phosphate related disorder. If a person has a deficiency in phosphate the failure of this enzymatic pathway would be expected. If G6P is not converted metabolically, then the body may request phosphate and glucose. This request for glucose would explain the "sweet tooth" the many bipolar people possess.

Atlanta pharmacist and doctor John S. Pemberton, as a nerve tonic, originally invented Coca-Cola. It is of note that Coca-Cola originally contained

---

[58] http://www.nimh.nih.gov/research/genetics.htm#gen12c

phosphate, carbonated water, sugar, and cocaine. This may have been a remedy devised for bipolar disease. I have wondered if Dr. Pemberton had been seeking a cure for bipolar disease. It is rumored that he died of kidney failure.

Phosphate contains phosphorus and oxygen. It is of supreme importance to humans because the body's energy comes from this source. Phosphate when released from the adenosine triphospate aka ATP yields energy. Phosphate provides energy for nearly all cell functions. Phosphate is also needed for red blood cells to release oxygen. In bipolar illness the kidney fails to reabsorb phosphate and energy levels are affected. **Low phosphate levels causes phosphate to move into cells activating an enzyme phosphofructokinase, which stimulates glycolysis.** This is probably stimulated by adenyl cyclase.

Glycolysis is defined as "The anaerobic enzymatic conversion of glucose to the simpler compounds lactate or pyruvate, resulting in energy stored in the form of adenosine triphosphate (ATP), as occurs in the muscle; it differs from respiration in that organic substances, rather than molecular oxygen, are used as electron acceptors." In order to fully convert one glucose molecule to ATP, we need magnesium in 12 of the 22 steps.

"The accelerated glycolysis of hypoxia serves as an alternative system for the generation of ATP when the normal mitochondrial mechanism is impaired."[59] Glycolysis is designed for the short run and it is not efficient, but possibly life saving. I believe a state of mild glycolysis exists in many "skinny" people that eat more than the average person.

Glycolysis leads to phosphate consumption. This creates a hyper catabolic state that worsens the condition. Any cause of hyperventilation can cause hypophoshatemia. Administering carbohydrate lowers serum phosphate by stimulating the release of insulin, which moves phosphate and glucose into cells.

This is what we see in bipolar patients. They crave sweets! Sugars are relatively simple organic compounds composed of carbon, hydrogen and oxygen. These are the same ingredients in the Henderson-Hasselbach equation. The metabolism of these sugars will be water and carbon dioxide. Hydrogen and bicarbonate are the intermediary ions. My theory is that the body realizes that the bicarbonate level is low and requests food to make this bicarbonate.

---

[59] Harrison's Principles of Internal Medicine, 10th Edition, page 680.

However, hydrogen ions are a byproduct. This makes the brewing acidosis worse. This increased amount of hydrogen causes even greater bicarbonate losses. Therefore, the additional request for sugar or refeeding.

Red blood cell function may be impaired because without phosphate the cells are fragile. The spleen destroys them. Tiredness is further increased by the failure of the red blood cell to release oxygen because of decreases in erythrocyte 2,3-DPG. So the **anemia** problem may not be so much with the production, but with the destruction of red blood cells. **Immunity** is affected because some white cells, responsible for killing bacteria and viruses, are not produced in sufficient quantities, especially the eosinophils.

Weakness is the most common symptom suggesting low phosphate levels. This may affect the eyes. Double vision may occur. Children may have for example **amblyopia**. The cause is from insufficient phosphate levels at the time of vision development.[60] The result is "weak eye". (I have this condition).

Cortisol, a glucocorticoid, is secreted normally twice a day. The times are usually 4 a.m. and 2 p.m. These are also periods of significant sleep. If you experience significant "afternoon swoon" your glucose 6-phosphate, manganese and chromium levels are probably low. Chromium improves glucose metabolism. When used with manganese, I have found chromium is useful in eliminating afternoon swoon.

So we see the bipolar description. This is a tired, thin person running late for work. He has some form of knock-knees or bowlegs or scoliosis or sunken chest and poor vision. He is having a bad hair day, eating sweets, and typically in a bad mood.

Phosphate has significant buffering capacity and it is the major buffer of renal solutions; that is, it can accept hydrogen ions. As a matter of fact, it can accept three hydrogen ions. The loss of phosphate with the reabsorption of chloride ion to maintain neutrality means that the ability to buffer acidity in the body is stressed. Therefore, excess hydrogen ion would exist.

Phosphate deficiency may result in glucose 6-phosphate deficiency. This may be involved in the sweet craving; that is, a deficiency in the substance glucose 6-phosphate causes a request for the ingredients to make this, glucose and phosphate. The body requests both and receives candy for glucose, but the continued

---

[60] http://www.emedicine.com/emerg/topic278.htm.

failure of phosphate reabsorption prevents adequate production. A deficiency in the substance Glucose 6-Phosphate is a cause of hemolytic anemia.

Respiratory alkalosis that is produced by compensation for metabolic acidosis causes increased respiration. Although this increased respiratory rate may go unnoticed it may be enough to activate the **enzyme phospho-fructokinase, which stimulates glycolysis.**[61] If the glycolysis is significant enough then weight loss may occur. This is probably the reason that many bipolar people are unusually lean. This characteristic is sometimes described as a failure to thrive.

Factors that promote phosphate deficiency include respiratory alkalosis, magnesium deficiency, and hyperparathyroidism.[62] All of these factors play significant parts in bipolar disease. Note that phosphate is actively reabsorbed via the sodium pump in the upper portion of the descending limb is sensitive to parathyroid hormone. It is possible that lower levels of phosphate may cause a decrease in phosphatidylserine that aids memory.

High Phosphate Content Foods

Wheat germ*
Peas*
Beans*
Lentils
Oats*
Cocoa beans
Tuna (note the possibility of mercury)
Liver
Mushrooms

Processed Foods High in Phosphate Content

Soft drinks (colas)
Chocolate
Ice cream

---

[61] Harrison's Principles of Internal Medicine, 10th Edition, page 679.
[62] http://www.ace.cc/electrolyte disturbances

Biscuits, cookies
Tomato ketchup
Mayonnaise
Processed cheese

GLYCOLYSIS ENERGY PRODUCTION

Glycolysis is a process in which glucose (sugar) is partially broken down by cells in enzyme reactions that do not need oxygen. Glycolysis is one method that cells use to produce energy. When glycolysis is linked with other enzyme reactions that use oxygen, more complete breakdown of glucose is possible and more energy is produced.[63]

Glycolysis is the making of molecules of the sugar, glucose. Glucose is manufacturer within the liver from fat or proteins. For example, amino acids, glycolysis intermediate molecules, or citric acid cycle intermediates may be used.[64]

Oxidative phosphorylation can only occur when the partial pressure of oxygen (PO_2) within the mitochondrion is above a critical level. Connett *et al* defined three theoretical thresholds of cell hypoxia. The first threshold is crossed when cell oxygen decreases but ATP production is maintained at a level sufficient to match ATP demand by metabolic adaptation. Adaptation involves recruitment of the redox component of electron transport, changes in the phosphorylation states of mitochondria, and increased glycolysis. The critical level of mitochondrial PO_2 for oxidative phosphorylation depends on the cells ability to adapt the phosphorylation process metabolically, and the level of ATP demand.

The second threshold occurs when steady state ATP turnover can only be maintained by supplementary production of ATP from anaerobic glycolysis, by the Embden-Meyerhof pathway. This energy inefficient mechanism for producing high-energy molecules generates only two molecules of ATP (67 kJ of available energy) for every molecule of glucose metabolised. The pathway must therefore either consume relatively larger quantities of glucose or, alternatively, yield much less ATP. *In high energy consuming organs, such as the brain, kidney, and liver, the rapid transfer of such quantities of glucose across cell membranes is not*

---

[63] http://hyperdictionary.com/search.aspx?define=glycolysis
[64] http://hyperdictionary.com/search.aspx?define=gluconeogenesis

possible. Therefore, these organs develop ATP depletion rapidly under hypoxic conditions. Dysoxia can be defined below the second threshold, where ATP production becomes oxygen limited. The third threshold is crossed when glycolysis becomes insufficient to produce enough ATP to maintain cell function and structural integrity.[65]

Cells require oxygen for the production of ATP, the principal energy source. ATP is hydrolysed to ADP and high-energy phosphate by adenosine triphosphatases in the cytosol. Energy released is used for the maintenance of membrane integrity, ionic pumps, and other specialised functions, such as contractility of muscle cells, and impulse transmission in neurons. The body's stores of ATP will last no more than a few minutes, so it must be synthesised continuously as it is being used. Under physiological conditions, most ATP is generated from the metabolism of glucose, by the process of oxidative phosphorylation.[66]

Cellular mitochondria perform oxidative phosphorylation. Oxidative phosphorylation requires the elements **iron and copper** to perform. The vitamins **niacin and riboflavin** are involved. **Hydrogen ions** are very involved in this pathway.[67] A nicely detailed explanation is available at the footnoted Website.

Thanks to Mrs. Sutera, a professor at Duke University, who wrote:

1ST step—(GLYCOLYSIS—splitting glucose):
Remember that you need to use energy to make energy. (*That's why you have to get yourself up and away for the TV—and out to get some exercise!!!* You will feel energized AFTER you have gone and expended some energy.) Therefore, the first step uses ATP to gain ATP.

$$C6H12O6 + 2\ ATP \text{------}> 2\ \textbf{pyruvic acid} + 4\ \textbf{ATP}$$

Pyruvic acid is simply half of a glucose molecule—we've chopped it in half. You made 4 molecules of ATP. Since you needed 2 molecules of ATP for the reaction, the <u>NET gain</u> is 2 ATP.

2nd step—the oxidation step:

$$\textbf{Pyruvic Acid} + O2 \text{------}> 34\ \textbf{ATP} + CO2 + H20$$

---

[65] http://adc.bmjjournals.com/cgi/content/full/archdischild%3b81/4/343

[66] http://adc.bmjjournals.com/cgi/content/full/archdischild%3b81/4/343

[67] http://www.sci.sdsu.edu/classes/biology/bio202/TFrey/OxidativePhos.html

Wow! When you add oxygen, the pyruvic acid molecule makes 34 ATP molecules. That's a lot of energy from a single glucose molecule! Those by-products of water and carbon dioxide diffuse out the cell and are carried away.

If you put steps 1 & 2 together, here's what you did:

$$C6H12O6 + 6\ O2 ------> 34\ ATP + 6\ CO2 + 6\ H2O$$

Some organisms don't use oxygen to make energy.

The first step of their respiration is GLYCOLYSIS (same as above). So they produce 2 ATP. Not much. Then again, yeast and bacteria don't need a whole lot of energy.

In their next step, they turn the pyruvic acid into 2 products we use in baking and brewing—carbon dioxide and alchohol!

Now—believe it or not, there is a time when humans undergo anaerobic **respiration**—it is when we work our muscles so hard that we deplete their oxygen supply. In this case, the pyruvic acid molecules don't turn into alcohol and carbon dioxide (otherwise you'd feel a little tipsy after exercise!). Instead, the pyruvic acid turns into something that makes your muscles sore. Lactic Acid![68]

ATP is considered the energetic currency of the cell, and it is centrally important in most energy requiring processes. At the cellular level thousands of individual reactions are involved in (1) energy transfer and (2) some energy loss (entropy factor =HEAT.) There are three types of energy sources (food) a. carbohydrates (sugars and glycogen) b. fats (fatty acids and glycerol, an alcohol) c. protein (strings of amino acids).

Food +O2+ADP P--->ATP +Heat +CO2.

ATP = ADP +P +energy (-7kcal)

Note the heat is produced. Do you remember our symptom of warm skin?

Note the carbon dioxide production. How does this interact with our carbonic anhydrase reaction? My expectation is that this CO2 is dissolved into cellular fluid as bicarbonate. This makes excess hydrogen ions available. Remember hydrogen ions equal acid.

---

[68] http://www.duke.edu/~djs3/bio/

Calcium loading causes a decrease in parathyroid hormone, which causes a decrease in phosphate excretion.[69] Negative inhibition of PTH release occurs primarily by direct effect of calcium at the level of the parathyroid gland. Although not well elucidated, 1,25-(OH)2 D3 appears to exert a mild inhibitory effect on the parathyroid gland as well.[70]

Frequent feeding may be caused from a **glucose 6-phosphate deficiency** which is probably caused from decreased phosphate reabsorption.[71] This may explain the sweet cravings.

Memory is associated with a compound known as phosphatidylserine. This is a phoshate compound. Obviously, a phosphate deficiency may wreak havoc with memory if the other systems are working properly.

Anemia derived from phosphate deficiency may occur in both the production and destruction of blood. In order to make hemoglobin the compound succinyl CoA required magnesium and phosphate to make hemoglobin.

---

[69] http://www.phys.mcw.edu/medphy/chout/lecture/lecture78

[70] http://www.emedicine.com/ent/topic539.htm

[71] Harrison's Principles of Internal Medicine, 10th Edition, page 1925

CHAPTER 15

Motion Sickness, Balance, Constipation, Explosive Diarrhea, and Grandiosity

The gyroscope ion, magnesium

I always had a knot on my head from where I had fallen; at least, that is what my Mom tells me. This may have been from magnesium deficiency creating *balance* difficulties. I can recall that in grade school the teacher had us walk a beam. I fell off, but many of my peers succeeded. I frequently had *motion sickness*. If my father did not pull the car to curb quickly it frequently meant cleaning up his car after I spewed. I remember as a child whirling around with other kids to get dizzy. However, I would be much more dizzy than them and the condition would last longer. Naturally, I did not like that feeling.

Even more disgusting than urine to talk about are bowel movements. Prior to starting this therapy my bowel movements were irregular. The stools were either small and pebble like or I had explosive diarrhea. The urge would hit at inopportune times and I would really have little control. For a period just the thought of going shopping was unpleasant because I did not know how my bowels were going to respond. Well, that all has changed. I now have regular and normal bowel movements. *My bowel movements are regular.*

My psychiatrist checked my peripheral temperature recently with a new gadget he had. My peripheral temperature was about 85. His was about 92. I believe this peripheral temperature tells you how well magnesium and phosphate are performing their basal energy duties.

I believe a discussion of bipolar disease would be incomplete without a discussion of grandiosity and suicide. I will attempt to provide a little insight into both topics although I have not researched either to a significant degree.

Grandiosity, as I see it, may be simply a symptom of unopposed nerve transmission. Simply put, grandiosity is an overactive imagination. I believe everyone has grandiose thoughts and expectations, or we would not have the popularity of the lottery or the success of shows like American Idol. Grandiosity becomes a problem when it crosses the line into the irrational. Magnesium plays a role in preventing excessive nerve transmission. We Americans tend to be deficient in magnesium. The treatment of grandiosity may just require normalization of magnesium levels. Suicide is covered in chapter 31.

I remember prior to being hospitalized with psychosis in 1991 that I had clumped this huge tapestry of vague associations together to weave some sort of grandiose world scheme. It's funny now, but the mind when it is not nourished properly will "play tricks on you". During this episode, this colossal scheme of vague associations seemed real, very real. Grandiosity that involves stress related images will certainly "rev-up" the adrenal system, which would promote psychosis.

My psychiatrist originally seeded my interest in magnesium 10 years earlier. He had interest in magnesium as a treatment for bipolar disorder. My thinking in developing this theory has been to accept what he sees and try to find a pathway to describe the symptoms or effects he identified. In this case, he was using magnesium chloride as the treatment. The problem with magnesium chloride is two fold, (1) the chloride ion probably causes nervousness and (2) the chloride ion may have contributed to acidosis thereby continuing the patient's trace element loss and preventing response. In investigating magnesium I found that it is a treatment for hyperparathyroidism. The article also included hypo parathyroid symptoms many of which corresponded to my complaints.

Functions of magnesium:
1. Energy cycles in glycolysis, magnesium is needed for 6 of 9 steps. In the citric acid cycle, it is needed in 4 out of 9 steps. In electron transport chain (cytochrome system) it is needed in 2 out of 4 steps. **So, to fully convert one glucose molecule to ATP, we need magnesium in 12 of the 22 steps.** (This conversion is probably inefficient due to lack of magnesium and phosphate. Therefore, basal energy will be low).
2. Liver function. Magnesium is involved in over 300 enzymes. Magnesium acts as a cofactor of glucuronyl transferase, which detoxifies estrogens. Magnesium is a co-factor for adenyl cyclase. **Magnesium is involved in all phosphorylases.** Magnesium enhances tryptophan hydroxylase. Magnesium is involved in the

production and utilization of DNA. Magnesium is necessary for muscle relaxation. **Low levels of magnesium may produce hypertension, asthma, cold hands/feet and headaches.** (An aside, I recently had the flu and my feet were very cold during this illness. Possibly the virus wreaks havoc with cellular magnesium metabolism). Magnesium may also produce poor muscle coordination, pupil size; peristalsis of colon needs coordinated muscle function (constipation), swallowing, and urine flow. Magnesium is required for production of neurotransmitter serotonin and melatonin; therefore, if the level of magnesium is low depression and sleep disturbances may result. Magnesium helps to control of blood sugar and it is needed for synchronous release of insulin for pancreas and gluconeogenesis. Magnesium is needed for antibody synthesis, voltage stability of nerve cells, protein synthesis and hemoglobin synthesis.[72]

Low levels of magnesium impair parathyroid hormone release, which blocks parathyroid hormone action on the bone. Lower parathyroid levels decrease the activity of 1 alpha hydroxylase, which activates vitamin D3. Magnesium deficiency impairs the intracellular transport of potassium and contributes to urinary wasting of potassium.[73]

Magnesium is an extremely important mineral. It is involved in over 300 metabolic reactions. Magnesium is required by ATP synthesizing protein in the mitochondria, the cellular powerhouse. Cell signaling requires MgATP for the phosphorylation, adding phosphate, of protein with formation of the cell signaling molecule cyclic AMP. Cyclic AMP causes an increase in production of parathyroid hormone. (Note that parathyroid hormone plays an important role in bipolar disease). Magnesium is required for nucleic acid synthesis, DNA and RNA, and protein. Magnesium is involved in carbohydrate and lipid synthesis.

Magnesium is involved in the synthesis of glutathione. (Note selenium is needed for glutathione peroxidase). **Magnesium is required for "active transport" of ions like potassium and calcium across cell membranes.** (This is important to people with bipolar disease because of the importance of preventing potassium and calcium depletion). Magnesium affects nerves impulses, muscle contractions and heart rhythm. Increased zinc ingestion produces decrease magnesium absorption. Ingestion of high amounts of protein causes decreased magnesium absorption.[74]

---

[72] http://www.jcem.endojournals.org/cgi/content/abstract/83/11/3857
[73] http://www.kidneyatlas.org/book1/adk1_04.pdf
[74] http://www.lpi.oregonstate.edu/infocenter/minerals.html

Glutamate is an amino acid that acts as an excitatory neurotransmitter. **Magnesium does inhibit the excitatory effect of glutamate.** "The excitatory amino acids <u>glutamate</u> (glu) and <u>aspartate</u> (asp) are thought to be the major excitatory transmitters. The inhibitory amino acids gamma-amino-butyric acid (GABA) and <u>glycine</u> (gly) are also essential for brain function

Magnesium is found in the extracellular fluid. When the membrane is polarized magnesium occupies its binding site and blocks the channel. This means that prolonged depolarization is needed to rid magnesium before glutamate can produce a flow of cations through the channel. There are two other sites that regulate the channel. At one zinc binds to block NMDA responses and at the other polyamines (spermine and spermidine) facititate NMDA transmission.[75] Note that the NMDA receptor is present in an inactive state with an Mg++ ion blocking the calcium channel. For the NMDA receptor to become active the Mg++ must leave the channel site. [76] Therefore, magnesium and zinc decrease excitation.

---

[75] http://www.psych.mcgill.ca/courses/522/UNIT7.htm
[76] http://www.dendrites.com/Trans95N.htm

CHAPTER 16

Sweaty Palms, Perspiration, Respiratory Infections, Skinny, and Warm Skin

Be a survivor-Your immunity card, zinc

I was *very skinny as a teenager* probably as a result of a hypercatabolic state developed from zinc deficiency. AS A SENIOR IN HIGH SCHOOL I WAS SIX FOOT THREE INCHES TALL AND I ONLY WEIGHED 155 POUNDS. I began having *frequent colds* around age 30. This was probably related to zinc defiency. One of my sons had their rate of metabolism checked in a biology experiment in school. The result was he had the highest rate of metabolism of anyone in the class. *Sweaty palms* are a symptom of zinc deficiency. When I played sports I would be drenched with sweat. I noticed that my friends did not *perspire heavily*.

Carbonic anhydrases are enzymes that catalyze the hydration of carbon dioxide and the dehydration of bicarbonate. These carbonic anhydrase driven reactions are of great importance in a number of tissues. Examples include:

- Parietal cells in the stomach secrete massive amounts of acid (i.e., hydrogen ions or protons) into the lumen and a corresponding amount of bicarbonate on into the blood.
- Pancreatic duct cells do essentially the opposite, with bicarbonate as their main secretory product.
- Secretion of hydrogen ions by the renal tubules is a critical mechanism for maintaining acid-base and fluid balance.
- Carbon dioxide generated by metabolism in all cells is removed from the body by red blood cells that convert most of it to bicarbonate for transport, and then back to carbon dioxide to be exhaled from the

lungs. Carbonic anhydrase isozymes are metalloenzymes consisting of a single polypeptide chain (Mr~29,000) complexed to an atom of zinc. They are incredibly active catalysts with a turnover rate (kcat) of about 1,000,000 reactions per second! Carbonic anhydrase inhibitors have been used therapeutically. The prototype of such drugs is acetazolamide, which is still sometimes used as a diruetic to treat certain edematous conditions and for therapy of some types of glaucoma. The discovery of this drug is actually an interesting story. It is a member of the sulfonamides, a group of antibacterial agents which, when initially investigated, were shown to induce a metabolic acidosis because they inhibited excretion of hydrogen ion from the kidney."[77] There are several very important factors that I found in this article. The most important though was the identification of zinc. Zinc is responsible for catalyzing this reaction. This helps prevent metabolic acidosis.

Parietal cells in the stomach secrete massive amounts of acid into the lumen and a corresponding amount of bicarbonate ion into the blood. Pancreatic duct cells do essentially the opposite, with bicarbonate as their main secretory product. Secretion of hydrogen ions by the renal tubules is a critical mechanism for maintaining acid/base and fluid balance. Carbon dioxide generated by metabolism in all cells is removed from the body by red blood cells that convert most of it to bicarbonate for transport, and then back to carbon dioxide to be exhaled from the lungs. (Carbonic anhydrase inhibitors such as acetazolamide produce symptoms of mental disease. If there is an excess of chloride ion, then an excess amount of acid may be produced. Bipolar patients tend to have lower amounts of red blood cells and, therefore, they may have more difficulty in eliminating carbon dioxide via respiration).

Secretion of hydrogen ion by tubular cells into lumen has an inverse relationship with potassium secretion.[78] In other words, the higher the potassium secretion the lower the hydrogen secretion.

It is the catalyst zinc that drives this reaction to neutral. If zinc is not sufficiently available, then too much hydrogen ion will exist producing acidity. In order to keep the body neutral, it is necessary to have enough bicarbonate or carbon dioxide to offset the hydrogen ion. Pancreatic secretions appear to have

[77] R. Bown, http://vivo.colostate.edu/hbooks/molecules/carbonic_anhydrase.html
[78] http://www.physiology.lsuhsc.edu/mgl/7.asp

high concentrations of zinc. Sweat contains approximately 1 mg zinc per liter. Normal urinary zinc ranges from 300 to 70mcg/24 hours. During stress, as much as 8000mcg zinc may be lost per day in the urine, primarily because of catabolism of skeletal muscle, which contains relatively high concentrations of zinc. **High urinary zinc excretion has been proposed as one indicator of a hyper catabolic state.**[79]

What stands out in this article is sweat. **An athlete is going to be very susceptible to acute zinc deficiency.** Also, the identification of hypercatabolic state is very important. Hypercatabolism means the body is breaking down too quickly; weight loss is the result. Biochemically, **zinc is essential for mobilization of vitamin A** from the liver. Zinc functions as an integral component of more than 70 known metalloenzymes through its involvement in protein, DNA and RNA synthesis. More than 90 percent of enzymatic zinc is present in the erythrocyte as carbonic anhydrase.

Night blindness can be a significant problem for bipolar patients. Zinc and vitamin A play critical roles in combating this problem. I also found the association between zinc and erythrocyte, red blood cells, fascinating.

The blood work of a bipolar patient will show low or low normal red blood cells. If a person who has too few red blood cells, then this anemia makes the possibility for metabolic acidosis, too much acid in the body, even greater.

Copper provides the catalytic activity for the antioxidant enzyme copper-zinc superoxide dismutase (CuZnSOD), while zinc plays a critical structural role. The structure and function of cell membranes are also affected by zinc. Loss of zinc from biological membranes increases susceptibility to oxidative damage and impairs their function.[80] Copper-zinc superoxide dismutase is a very potent anti-oxidant. Zinc also plays a role in cell signaling and has been found to influence hormone release and nerve impulse transmission.[81]

The symptoms of severe zinc deficiency include the slowing or cessation of growth and development, delayed sexual maturation, characteristic skin rashes, chronic and severe diarrhea, immune system deficiencies, impaired wound healing, diminished appetite, night blindness, and behavior disturbances.[82]

---

[79] http://surgery.mc.duke.edu/nutrition/secure/trace_elements.html.

[80] http://www.lpi.oregonstate.edu/infocenter/minerals.html

[81] http://www.lpi.oregonstate.edu/infocenter/minerals.html

[82] http://www.lpi.oregonstate.edu/infocenter/minerals.html

"…Preliminary evidence indicates that sexual maturation, growth, and development depend on adequate dietary zinc."[83] High amounts of zinc are found in bones, teeth, hair, skin, liver, muscle, and testes. About 1/3 is loosely bound to the protein albumin and 2/3 are firmly bound to globulins. Zinc is present in red blood cells mainly as part of the enzyme carbonic anhydrase. Signs of deficiency are poor appetite, poor growth, impaired taste, and hypogonadalism. **Hepatic encephalopathy responds to zinc probably through improved enzymatic conversion of ammonia to urea.**[84] Note that the glutamine pathway produces excess ammonia. Zinc probably helps eliminate neuro-toxic ammonia which has been implicated in **attention** disorders.

Sweat contains approximately 1mg of zinc per liter. This makes **athletes especially vulnerable zinc deficiency** and possibly above average pH levels, that is, more acidic. During stress as much as 8000mcg of zinc may be lost per day in urine. The primary reason is because of catabolism of skeletal muscle, which contains high concentrations of zinc. High urinary zinc excretion is an indicator of a hyper catabolic state. Zinc is essential for vitamin A. More than 90 percent of enzymatic zinc is present in the erythrocyte as carbonic anhydrase. Zinc is helpful in healing surgical wounds. Deficiency can produce anorexia and weight loss. [85]

Zinc is involved in the important enzyme CuZnSOD or copper zinc super oxide dimutase. Zinc appears to be involved in gene directed cell death.

The absorption of a mineral is affected by other minerals.
- The presence of iron in the gut may decrease zinc absorption
- The presence of zinc in the gut may decrease copper absorption
- The presence of calcium in the gut may decrease zinc absorption
- The presence of zinc in the gut increases folic acid absorption.

Zinc has 3 primary roles:
  (1) Catalytic expression involves
      (a) Over 100 enzymes
      (b) Structural
      (c) Regulatory

---

[83] Harrison's Principles of Internal Medicine, 10th Edition, page 471
[84] Merck Manual, Fifteenth Edition, 1987, page 839
[85] http://surgery.mc.duke.edu/nutrition/secure/trace_elements.html.

(2) Regulatory expression involves
    (a) Gene expression transcription factor
    (b) Cell signaling hormone release

Recent research indicates zinc availability affects cell-signaling systems that coordinate the response to the **growth-regulatory hormone, and insulin-like growth factor.** Lower maternal zinc causes diminished attention of newborn and poorer motor function at 6 months.

There is a high concentration of zinc in the retina. Retinal zinc declines with age and it may produce age related macular degeneration. [86]

Food sources include *oysters, crab, beef, pork, turkey, yogurt, cheese, milk, cashews, almonds, peanuts, and beans. The recommended daily allowance of zinc in an adult woman is 8 mg and 11 mg in adult men.[87] **It cannot be stressed enough that in the bipolar person that zinc is very important to maintaining neutralizing acidosis.**

Zinc is found in high concentrations in secretions (tears, saliva, sweat, gastric acid, intestinal fluid, and synovial fluid. lubricant and antiseptic to clean off pathogenic organisms from body surface). Low zinc levels may cause dry mouth, dry vagina, sore throats, and mouth ulcers. Low levels of zinc affect the immune system, which require zinc for white cell production. Zinc is necessary for tissue repair; therefore, low zinc levels may delay wound healing. Zinc is necessary for the function of enzymes alcohol dehydrogenanse and alkaline phosphatase (typically low in bipolar patients). Zinc is involved with **steroid hormone production** and insulin production.

Zinc is necessary for the senses of taste & smell, the biochemistry of vision, & normal function of nerves; necessary for brain development, & for adult brain function; Zn-deficient brain cells shrink; [88]

---

[86] http://www.lpi.oregonstate.edu/infocenter/minerals.html
[87] http://www.lpi.oregonstate.edu/infocenter/minerals.html
[88] http://www.enerex.ca/nutrition_digest_book.htm#Bb11

CHAPTER 17

Body Heat and Anxiety

"Jimmy Buffer" the outside world

When I was a child I heard about a gentleman who died of a heart attack. The adults who were talking about it said that the death was blamed on "bicarb." We know that as bicarbonate of soda or baking soda. I had a headache one day last year so I tried an Alka-Seltzer that we had in the pharmacy. This product contained sodium bicarbonate and acetaminophen. I had never previously tried Alka-Seltzer. I was amazed at this feeling. I could feel my body cool and I became calmer.

The *runny nose* symptom began after I age 35. It, however, became annoying. I suspect that runny nose is another symptom for acidosis. Since beginning this therapy the frequency, duration, and quantity has diminished dramatically.

What causes *body heat*? Body heat is directly related to acidity in the body. Heat is created when a chemical reaction produces energy. These are called exothermic reactions. It is common for reactions that produce acids to produce heat energy. It is a simple chemical equation.

$$CO_2 \text{ (gas phase)} \Longleftrightarrow CO_2 + H_2O \Longleftrightarrow H_2CO_3 \Longleftrightarrow H^+ + HCO_3^-$$

(In this condition, metabolic acidosis, the excess hydrogen ions push the carbonic reaction from above to the left to eliminate CO_2. This excess CO_2 causes an increase in respiration.)[89]

---

[89] Modified from http://www.physiology.lsuhsc.edu/mgl/mgl7.asp

In this sequence water, H20, must be split, H20 $<==>$ H+ + OH-. I believe this reaction proceeds with the help of the enzymes known as hydroxylases and dehydrogenases. My theory establishes 1-alpha hydroxylase is affected and that another hydroxylase enzyme, which is known as 7-alpha hydroxylase, fails as well. This may be a phenomenon where some, most, or all hydroxylase enzymes are affected to some degree. Note, too, that the volume of water in the bipolar person may be less if the level of ADH, antidiuretic hormone, is low. Once the water is split then the reaction with carbon dioxide, CO2, may occur. However, in people with bipolar disease, I theorize, the enzyme carbonic anhydrase II is not available in sufficient quantity or the enzyme does not function properly due to a 1,25 DHCC deficiency that prevents it's expression. So, we are left with excess H+ and excess OH-. Hydroxide, also know as OH-, is very reactive toward strong positive ions. Therefore alkali such as calcium, potassium, magnesium, etc. would be expected to bind this ion. These compounds are basic and this probably explains the alkaline urine in RTA.[90]

---

[90] www.pubmedcentral.nih.gov.1992 The National Academy of Sciences, 1 alpha, 25 vitamin D3

CHAPTER 18

Sadness, Seasonal Affective Disorder, Afternoon Swoon, and Prolonged Bleeding

The way to avoid a "blue, blue, blue Christmas, Elvis"

Obviously I cannot see myself unless I look in the mirror, but prior to this therapy people would frequently say, "smile." I did not realize that I wasn't smiling. There are several factors that may participate in this smile, but probably it is GABA related. Anyway, *I seem to smile a more frequently.*

I had always been significantly affected by the changing of the seasons, especially going from summer to fall and winter to spring. This is known as seasonal affective disorder. This condition is common in the bipolar community. When my son was in the hospital a counselor mentioned that a bipolar colleague of hers used full spectrum UV lighting to control the seasonal affective disorder and even his bipolar condition. This piqued my interest so I researched this area. I found some are high UV states, such as California and Hawaii, and low UV states, such as Vermont and West Virginia.[91] I knew that manganese was a light sensitive mineral. I had purchased eyeglasses years earlier known as "photo gray extras" that contained manganese. In sunlight these eyeglasses darkened and in room light these lenses would return to a normal

---

91 www.national weather service

clear glass. I found out that through research that manganese was found in high concentrations in the eye. I learned that manganese was also involved in converting glutamate to GABA.

These sequences of events led me to a little experiment with my son. I had learned that black tea contained significant amounts of manganese and magnesium. I made "sun tea" as he went for a short walk. Then we sat on the deck drinking the tea in the summer sun. To my amazement his dilated eyes returned to normal. Even with the medicine he was taking prescribed by the psychiatrists this had not occurred. This initial reaction spurred me forward to other experiments. If I had not met with success here I may not have pursued the other tests.

Manganese seems to be the ion needed for proper awakening, the human alarm clock. My awakening used to be very erratic. Sometimes I would awaken at 5 a.m. and the next day it would be 10:30 a.m. before I arose. Now, I awaken at 6:15 in the morning without the alarm clock. It's nice to be on time for work rather than hurrying out the door trying to tie my tie and open the car door at the same time.

Afternoon swoon is a term I use to describe the extremely tired and sleepy feeling I used to get around 2 p.m. I could take a siesta in a heartbeat at that time of the day. I no longer experience that effect. I believe manganese along with chromium helps to prevent this symptom.

This year I have not experienced season affective disorder. I have experienced this condition as long as I can remember. Manganese is a cofactor in activating enzymes known as hydrolases, kinases, **decarboxylases** and tranferases. Manganese is important in the bone formation, energy production, protein, and fat metabolism. Manganese is necessary for mitochondria, the powerhouse where ATP is made. Manganese is found to play part in the formation of thyroxine, the active principle of the secretion of thyroid gland.[92] Manganese is a key component of the superoxide dismutase found in mitochondria of the cells. Without MnSOD an accumulation of free radicals would lead to severe membrane damage. [93]Manganese is important in building and breakdown cycles of protein and nucleic acids. **A manganese deficiency is shown to reduce the clotting response of vitamin K.** (Bruising or bleeding

---

[92] http://www.lpi.oregonstate.edu/infocenter/minerals.htmlhttp://
www.lpi.oregonstate.edu/infocenter/minerals.html

[93] A review from the Literature by Tuula E. Tuormaa for FORESIGHT, the Association for the Promotion of Preconceptual Care.
First published in: Journal of Orthomolecular Medicine, 11(3): 69-79, (Sept. 1996)

may be a symptom of manganese deficiency. I experienced this). Manganese stimulates adenylate cyclase activity in the brain. Cyclic AMP has a regulatory role in the action of several brain neurotransmitters (second messenger). **Manganese is a potent stimulator of adenyl cyclase activity whereas lead, mercury, zinc, and copper are powerful inhibitors of the enzyme.**[94]

Manganese is found in skeleton, liver, kidney, pancreas, and heart. Manganese absorption negatively affected by copper, zinc, cobalt, phosphorus, and calcium as well as soy protein. It is important to remember that amalgam fillings contain mercury and that bipolar people tend to have many fillings due to bone weakness and sweet craving. Therefore, it may be wise to take manganese on an empty stomach or with lecithin (chocolate is a source of lecithin). <u>Choline (eggs) and ethanol enhances intestinal uptake.</u> Manganese is excreted in bile. About 4 or 5 mg is accepted as RDA. Foods that contain significant amounts of manganese include tea, nuts, whole grains, spices and legumes. Manganese is necessary for chondroitin sulfate synthesis. This is important in arthritis type conditions. [95]

Manganese is involved in glucose metabolism. **Lower blood levels of manganese are found in epileptic patients. Some psychiatrists believe that this disease is similar to seizure disorders and this may be the reason.** Severely deficient manganese causes decreased libido. The western diet tends to be deficient because the most frequently eaten foods such as meat, fish and dairy which only have traces of manganese. Soil treated with agrochemicals is low in manganese. Liming the soil causes manganese depletion. Therefore, it may be necessary to take a manganese supplement because of insufficient manganese in the food supply. Foetal manifestations of manganese deficiency includes skeletal and cartilage abnormalities, defective skull and otolish, ataxia, lipid and carbohydrate metabolism defects and depressed reproduction function.[96]

Manganese is a mineral that acts as a **co-factor to the vitamins pyridoxine, panto-thenic acid, and biotin.** High concentrations are found in the brain, kidney, pancreas, liver and bones. Stimulating DNA and RNA synthesis involve manganese in protein synthesis. Manganese is involved in bone development. Manganese is involved in chondroitin sulfate synthesis. Chondroitin sulfate

---

[94] A review from the Literature by Tuula E. Tuormaa for FORESIGHT, the Association for the Promotion of Preconceptual Care.

First published in: Journal of Orthomolecular Medicine, 11(3): 69-79, (Sept. 1996)

[95] A review from the Literature by Tuula E. Tuormaa for FORESIGHT, the Association for the Promotion of Preconceptual Care.

[96] Journal of Orthomolecular Medicine, 11(3): 69-79, (Sept. 1996).

may be effective in some forms of arthritis. Manganese is helpful in wound healing for collagen production. Manganese is eliminated via the GI tract via bile and pancreatic juices. Manganese deficiency may express marked hypo-cholesterolemia.[97] Manganese is necessary for Manganese super oxide dimutase, MnSOD. Manganese is involved in gluconeogenesis with pyridoxine. Deficiency can change hair color. Deficiency can slow hair growth. Iron may decrease absorption of manganese. Signs of deficiency include decreased growth, decreased reproduction, abnormal skeleton, impaired glucose tolerance (note chromium is involved with glucose tolerance factor), and altered carbohydrate metabolism. Sources of manganese include pineapple, pecans almonds, cashews, peanuts, *Raisin Bran Cereal, bread beans, spinach, and tea.[98] (My cholesterol and my sister's cholesterol has been low in our past tests. My sister's was extremely low).

The concentration of manganese per gram dry tissue weight was determined in samples from 39 areas of 8 normal human brains. Manganese was shown to be unevenly distributed with the largest concentrations in the pineal gland and the olfactory bulb. The gray matter yielded a higher content of manganese than the white matter. Significant differences between individuals were found for identical areas of the gray and white matter of the cerebral cortex.[99]

Low levels of manganese in the body can contribute to infertility, bone malformation, weakness, and seizures. Manganese deficiencies are considered rare, however, since it is relatively easy to obtain adequate amounts of manganese through the diet. Interestingly, though, some experts estimate that as many as 37% of Americans do not get the recommended daily amounts of manganese in their diet. This may be due to the fact that whole grains are a major source of dietary manganese, and many Americans consume refined grains more often than whole grains. Refined grains provide half the amount of manganese as whole grains. Diseases associated with manganese deficiency are osteoporosis, diabetes, arthritis, epilepsy, pre-menstrual syndrome, and dysfunctional muscle co-ordination. [100]

---

[97] http://surgery.mc.duke.edu/nutrition/secure/trace_elements.html.

[98] http://www.lpi.oregonstate.edu/infocenter/minerals.html

[99] http://www.ncbi.nlm.nih.gov/entrez/query.fcgi?cmd=Retrieve&db= PubMed&list_uids=7121709&dopt=AbstractPMID: 7121709 [PubMed—indexed for MEDLINE]

[100] http://www.umm.edu/altmed/ConsSupplements/Manganesecs.html

URO-BILIARY PSYCHOSIS PATHWAY

1 alpha hydroxylase failure in kidney
◆
Active vitamin D failure; 1,25 dihydroxycholecalciferol
◆
Low phosphate levels, hypophosphatemia
◆
Sweet craving stimulated
◆
Glycolysis stimulated
◆
Attention deficits

Bicarbonate reabsorption fails, excess chloride ion reabsorbed.

7 alpha hydroxylase down-regulates bile metabolism resulting in mineral losses of copper and manganese	Hyperchloremic metabolic acidosis increases urinary excretion of calcium, magnesium, zinc, cobalt and iron

Stress stimulates cortisol synthesis

Cortisol inhibits active vitamin D synthesis

Increased mineral losses with excess chloride ion

PSYCHOSIS

CHAPTER 19

Insomnia Terror and Tremors

"To die, to sleep, perchance to dream"

I hated the *insomnia*. I had anxiety over the anticipation of bedtime. At night I could not fall asleep unless I was watching Good Will Hunting or Bull Durham. The anxiety and terror of the possibility of sleep induction failure was tremendous. Night after night, I would lie on the couch hoping for sleep. I knew sleep would not follow, which led to sleep anxiety. I had grown accustomed to using clonazepam, an antianxiety medicine, to help me fall asleep. Now, I take an absorbable copper supplement with thiamine and pyridoxine and I sleep like a baby. *My sleep is normal.*

I was still pursuing my understanding of sleep initiation and found, **"Copper is a functional part of the enzyme tyrosinase, which is essential for conversion of tyrosine to melanin."**[101] Tyrosinase is a copper monooxygenase that catalyzes the *hydroxylation* of monophenols and diphenols.[102]

```
                                         Vitamin C, copper
            Phenylalanine hydroxylase        tyrosine hydroxylase
Phenylalanine-------------------------->tyrosine ---------------------------->dopa


Dopa decarboxylase                  dopamine hydroxylase
--------------------------->dopamine ----------------------------->norepinephrine[103]
Vitamin B-6
                    (controls tremors)
```

Modified by d.m.

---

[101] http://surgery.mc.duke.edu/nutrition/secure/trace_elements.html.

[102] http://pfam.wustl.edu/cgi-bin/getdesc?acc=PF00264

[103] http://www.sbuniv.edu/~ggray.wh.bol/CHE3364/b1c25out.html

I had been concerned about my son's inability to fall asleep. The information I researched from Roche Biomedical showed that copper was involved in the reactions of converting melanin to melatonin. I had my son try copper at bedtime. He did sleep better. But what was amazing was that his essential tremor, which he had always had, went away. No tremor, wow! Now we had 3 elements that were deficient, all cations. I began to ask myself why cations? There were only three methods I knew of that could effect blood levels of those ions (1) nutritional ingestion deficiency, (2) malabsorption of nutrition, and (3) excessive excretion via the kidney. I knew number one could not be a factor because food was available and although his appetite was not the best, he did eat. Number two was ruled out because he had no stomach ailment or complaint. So I concentrated on number three, excessive excretion.

I had identified manganese, zinc, copper, and magnesium as deficiencies. I concluded that something was causing pan-cation loss. What could cause this? Ingestion? No, I ate very well, perhaps, better than my friends that I characterized as normal, (2) malabsorption, although I had diarrhea occasionally it was not frequent enough to significantly effect nutrition, however, (3) increased excretion seemed to be the best solution. "Which form of excretion?" was the next question. There are two primary forms of excretion, the intestines via biliary secretion and the kidneys. The kidneys seemed more logical since we were talking about mineral ions. At this point I decided to learn what I could about the kidneys. I had a medical text, Harrison's Principles of Internal Medicine, that I had since I graduated from pharmacy school. I rarely used it, but in the next few weeks Harrison's became my friend. I reviewed the chapter on kidney disease. I came to one disease that I that was completely unknown to me, distal renal tubular acidosis. I made the connection between acidosis and kidney.

In the meantime, I had been trying to find the element that may produce awakening. I had found that tryptophan is converted to serotonin, which is converted to melatonin. Serotonin is the substance that Prozac enhances. Prozac is related to the amphetamine class of drugs. Hence, I surmised that serotonin must be the "up and Adam" substance.

The morning awakening process seems to involve at least three items (1) cortisol which begins to be produced at about 4 a.m., (2) serotonin, and (3) UV light which stimulated the retina. Remember that manganese is light sensitive and it is also necessary for the conversion of alpha ketoglutamine to GABA. I found, however, that chromium was the necessary catalyst for the conversion of melatonin to serotonin or down-regulates melatonin synthesis. Cortisol's actions are probably tied to its mineralocorticoid effect. It probably raises the levels of these minerals slightly to stimulate enzymatic reactions necessary to produce awakening. I tried chromium on myself and it worked!

My trial with my son turned out to work, but I learned that you do not want to awaken an "angry bear." Meaning, before using chromium in therapy it is wise to let the patient "hibernate" because it is an efficient way to restore the minerals and, therefore, the mood.

All of a sudden I had a treatment and it worked. Yet, it did not completely explain what was happening. My son was a difficult patient so I continued trying to find a palatable liquid nutritional solution that would supplement the trace elements. I found a product that seemed to supply all the answers. It is called Boost and manufactured by Mead Johnson. We continued to have milk in the refrigerator and now Boost. However, he did not seem to be doing as well on Boost as he was on the cashews. I wondered, "Why"? One night while I was reading I came across, much by accident, hypervitaminosis D. I read the symptoms. They were anorexia, frequent urination, frequent thirst, weakness, nervousness, itching, and nausea and vomiting. They struck a bell.

After calculating my approximate vitamin D intake I realized this was a problem. I deleted Boost and milk from our refrigerator. I knew, however, that supplementing calcium would be a problem. I had to find a good calcium source. I found Tums, calcium carbonate, to be excellent. There is evidence that lithium decreases calcium urinary excretion and lithium carbonate is the only form of lithium that works. This may partially explain some of the effectiveness that lithium exhibits in treating bipolar disease.

I kept reviewing information on calcium, vitamin D, and the kidney. I found myself reading about the macula densa portion of the kidney and phosphate reabsorption failure. I learned that 1,25 DHCC was necessary for calcium and phosphate reabsorption. I knew there was a prescription form of 1,25 DHCC known as "Rocaltrol," which was used in treatment of kidney disease. At my August appointment with my psychiatrist I gave him a brief explanation of what I thought was causing this disease. These visits are brief and the information I gave him was substantial. For the first time he complimented me on my appearance. He said, "Keep doing what you are doing."

I explained to him that I thought this involved only the distal tubule and in my case only one kidney. I explained further that I didn't know if that would work necessarily because only one kidney was affected. In any case, he did not give me a prescription for Rocaltrol. I went back home and reviewed some more web sites. I went to emedicine and searched hypoparathyroid treatment. I found another answer! **Calcium loading stimulates the production of parathyroid hormone, which stimulates the production of 1,25 DHCC.** This stimulates gastro-intestinal phosphate absorption.

"Calcium?" I thought. The answer was again Tums. I understood also that the carbonate portion of this molecule would be converted in the body to bicarbonate. I went to my local drugstore and purchased Tums. I had had a raspy voice, which I had theorized was a symptom. My hypothesis was that by taking six Extra Strength Tums, equivalent to 2 grams of calcium, my parathyroid hormone would be stimulated and my voice would be normal. In the morning I awoke to a resonant deep voice. "This worked!"

Note too the similarity of CaCO3 (calcium carbonate) and LiCO3 (lithium carbonate). Both items provide carbonate, which can be converted to bicarbonate in the stomach by accepting a hydrogen ion that is readily available in stomach acid. Also, both have an effect on calcium metabolism. Calcium directly and lithium by decreasing urinary calcium excretion.[104]

---

[104] http://www.endocrinology.med.ucla.edu/hypercalcemia.htm

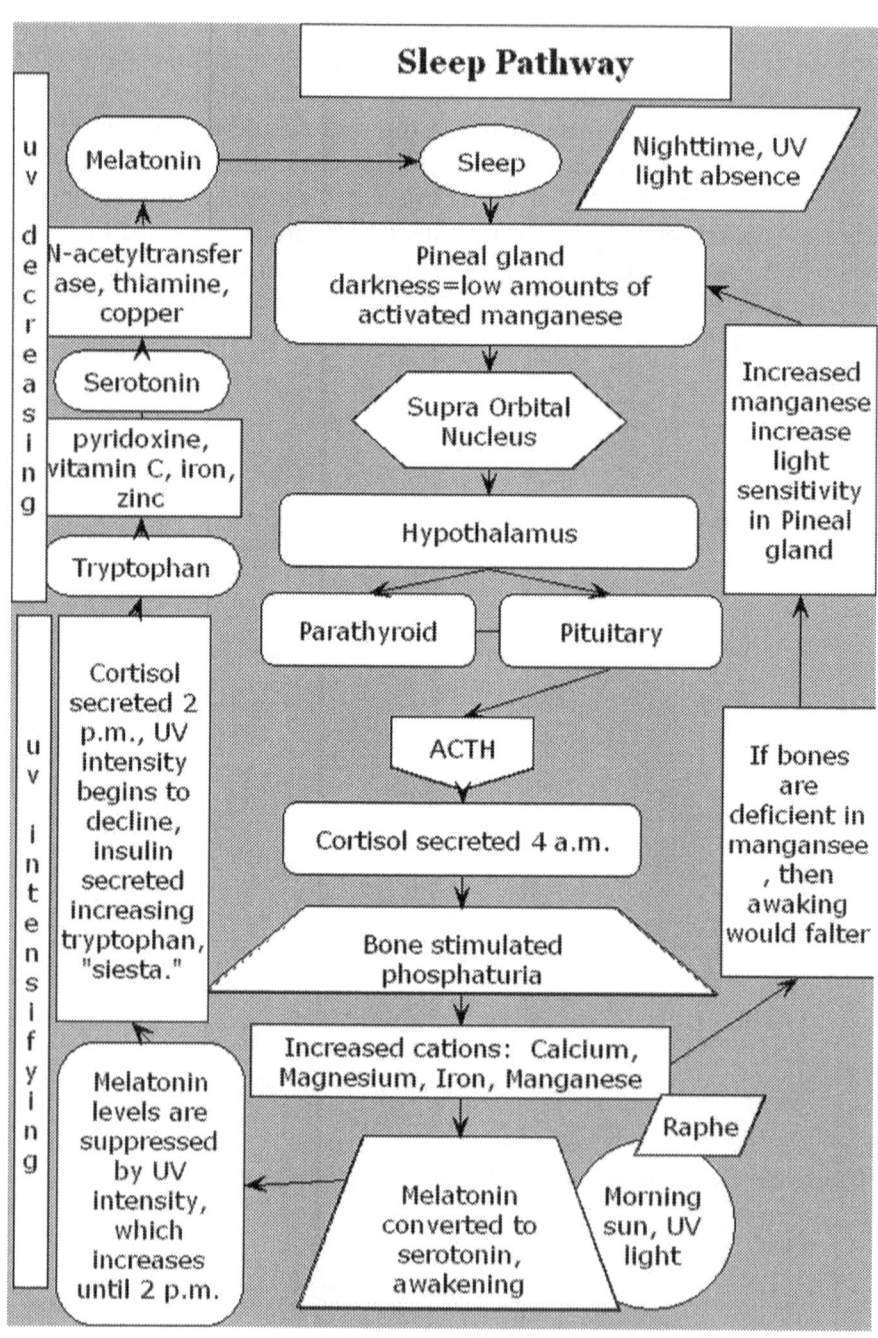

Sleep Pathway

uv decreasing

Melatonin → Sleep

Nighttime, UV light absence

N-acetyltransferase, thiamine, copper

Pineal gland darkness=low amounts of activated manganese

Serotonin

Supra Orbital Nucleus

pyridoxine, vitamin C, iron, zinc

Increased manganese increase light sensitivity in Pineal gland

Tryptophan

Hypothalamus

Parathyroid   Pituitary

uv intensifying

Cortisol secreted 2 p.m., UV intensity begins to decline, insulin secreted increasing tryptophan, "siesta."

ACTH

If bones are deficient in mangansee, then awaking would falter

Cortisol secreted 4 a.m.

Bone stimulated phosphaturia

Increased cations: Calcium, Magnesium, Iron, Manganese

Melatonin levels are suppressed by UV intensity, which increases until 2 p.m.

Raphe

Melatonin converted to serotonin, awakening

Morning sun, UV light

CHAPTER 20

Cramping, Frequent Urination and Excessive Thirst

Orange juice daily

I have experienced severe leg cramps in the past. I could also drink enormous quantities of liquid. Prior to becoming psychotic back in 1991 I recall I had to go to the restroom very frequently. *I now drink orange juice daily and I have not experienced cramping or urinary symptoms.*

Potassium is an anion found predominantly inside the cell. It is necessary to have adequate quantities within the cell so that the cell may work properly. Serum potassium may be significantly affected by a decline in bicarbonate or zinc concentration. A decline of either may result in more acidic pH levels. **Metabolic acidosis causes an increased movement for intracellular to extra cellular fluids. This movement results in higher urinary potassium loss.** Alkalosis, more basic, produces the opposite effect of extra cellular potassium moving intracellular. A small change in pH of 0.1 unit results in a 0.6 mEq/liter change in serum potassium. Severe hypokalemia causes muscle weakness, hypoventilation (which may produce glycolysis) and paralytic ileus (constipation).

It is important to note that potassium nephropathy produces the same symptoms as vitamin D toxicity. Those symptoms are polyuria and secondary polydipsia, frequent urination and frequent fluid intake or thirst. Does this mean that vitamin D toxicity produces potassium loss?

Bicarbonate is neutralized by excess calcium and other cations. Hydrogen is not secreted via the Na/H pump effectively. (Does the pump fail because of deficiency of phosphate, magnesium or both?) The net results are alkali carbonates being excreted in the urine or deposited in the kidney where they can do damage. Vitamin C is a urinary acidifier. By acidifying the urine more bicarbonate can be reabsorbed. How does vitamin C acidify the urine? If it is supposed to increase hydrogen ion secretion via the Na/H pump and this pump is not working properly, then this will only increase acidosis. Zinc is a cofactor of carbonic anhydrase. Zinc is necessary for conversion of neutral bicarbonate to hydrogen ion and bicarbonate ion in the renal tubular cells. Bicarbonate ion is reabsorbed and hydrogen ion is secreted in to renal lumen via the Na/H pump. If the zinc level were low, then the quantity of hydrogen ion available to be secreted would be low as well as bicarbonate to be reabsorbed. Further, the Na/K pump, which require magnesium because it is an ATP pump, of the interstitial cells works normally reabsorbing sodium and moving potassium into the tubular cells. Because of the low levels of hydrogen ions in the tubular cells, potassium takes the place of some hydrogen ions and it is secreted into the renal lumen. The consequence of this sequence is potassium is wasted.

CHAPTER 21

Caffeine Sensitivity

Just one cup please

Molydenum is responsible for activating the enzyme xanthine oxidase. An example of a xanthine is caffeine. This is the enzyme responsible for breaking down caffeine. A person with too liitle of this enzyme would be extremely sensitive to the effects of coffee. People with insomnia will very likely drink coffee and, probably, in high quantities in order that they make perform normal daily duties. The effects of drinking a cup of coffee will last much longer than a normal person. This obviously makes the insomnia much worse. Personally, I experienced this effect.

Molybdenum acts as a cofactor for riboflavin[105] Bipolar people may be more sensitive to effects of coffee because of a deficiency of molydenum.

---

[105] http://www.medscape.com/content/1996/00/40/88/408813/408813_tab.html

CHAPTER 22

Glucose Intolerance

Stress identifier

The mineral chromium absorbed from foodstuffs (not the Erin Brockovich type of chromium) is involved with a metabolic complex known as GLUCOSE TOLERANCE FACTOR or GTF for short. GTF helps insulin transfer sugar into the cells where the sugar can be used. Chromium, however, is excreted through the kidneys. This is the element that gives urine an orange tint. Since chromium is lost via the urine, metabolic acidosis will increase chromium excretion. This may be a way to identify the beginning of stress. Therefore, simply by noticing the change in your urine color you can identify a stress related event that is producing physical change. A chromium deficiency may make you prone to acidosis because a decrease in GTF will result in decreased sugar metabolism efficiency. If coupled with an increase in carbohydrate consumption an increase in lactic acid is the most likely result.

Commonly, increased carbohydrate consumption does occur during stress. Stress produces increased levels of cortisol, which inhibits 1 alpha hydroxylase. The result is excessive phosphate loss and, therefore, energy loss. A decrease, I believe, in glucose 6-phosphate would occur. This would result in glucose and phosphate craving.

Chromium is necessary for glucose tolerance factor. Chromium helps normalize glucose utilization by increasing peripheral tissue sensitivity to insulin. Therefore, a color change in urine to orange coupled with increased carbohydrate craving signifies stress is affecting the body. By knowing this bipolar people can take steps to eliminate the stressor.

A good sign of determining stress is sweaty palms. I have found that you can identify a person who is under stress by shaking their hand. A person who is under stress will have sweaty palms. I was speaking to a salesman once who was trying to sell me a condominium. I shook his hand before he began making his presentation. His hand at that time was sweaty. I shook his hand at the end of the presentation and his hand was normal. Obviously, he was experiencing consider-able stress during this time. Attention parents, shake you sons and daughters hands from time to time. If they are under stress, please find out why.

If necessary, please seek the appropriate help. As you will learn under the topic of suicide, it could mean the difference between life and death.

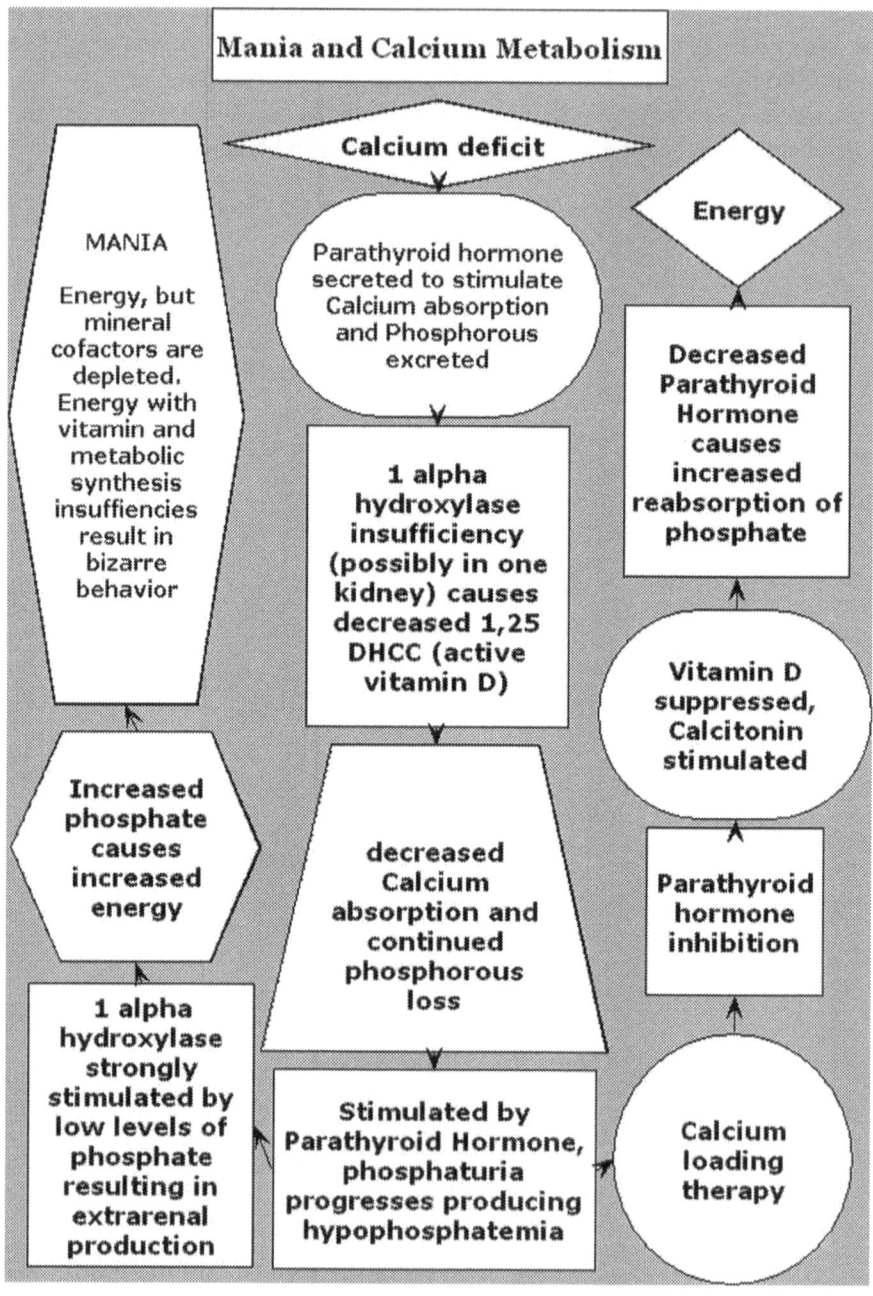

Mania and Calcium Metabolism

Calcium deficit

Energy

MANIA

Energy, but mineral cofactors are depleted. Energy with vitamin and metabolic synthesis insuffiencies result in bizarre behavior

Parathyroid hormone secreted to stimulate Calcium absorption and Phosphorous excreted

Decreased Parathyroid Hormone causes increased reabsorption of phosphate

1 alpha hydroxylase insufficiency (possibly in one kidney) causes decreased 1,25 DHCC (active vitamin D)

Vitamin D suppressed, Calcitonin stimulated

Increased phosphate causes increased energy

decreased Calcium absorption and continued phosphorous loss

Parathyroid hormone inhibition

1 alpha hydroxylase strongly stimulated by low levels of phosphate resulting in extrarenal production

Stimulated by Parathyroid Hormone, phosphaturia progresses producing hypophosphatemia

Calcium loading therapy

CHAPTER 23

Tired and Anemic

"The Ironman, Ozzie"

I don't know, but I suspect that Ozzie has bipolar disease. He has many of the symptoms like balance problems and drinking excessively. He is "artsy" like many bipolar people. Obviously, over the years his behavior has been very erratic. I notice he is consuming large quantities of nutritional supplements, which may be helpful if used correctly. So if anyone reads this book and they know Ozzie, then let him know about this book.

A few years ago I had some blood work and I was informed my hemoglobin was low. In addition over the years I have experienced some restless leg syndrome. Both of these conditions are associated with iron deficiency.

Iron is necessary to form hemoglobin, the oxygen carrier of the red blood cell. Deficiency produces anemia. Deficiency also may decrease cellular immunity and decrease bactericidal leukocytes (white cells). Tea forms insoluble iron tannate complexes, which prevent absorption. Iron is normally absorbed with difficulty and most people barely meet daily requirements. [106] A decrease in vitamin A may worsen iron deficiency anemia. [107] **Copper is required for iron transport to bone marrow for red blood cell formation.** Ingesting high amount of iron decreases zinc absorption. Ingesting high amount of calcium causes decrease iron absorption. Athletes' losses of iron are greater than the average person and may produce increased lead levels. Iron deficiency may produce restless leg syndrome.[108] **Iron**

[106] Merck Manual, Fifteenth Edition, 1987, page 942

[107] http://www.lpi.oregonstate.edu/infocenter/minerals.html

[108] http://www.lpi.oregonstate.edu/infocenter/minerals.html

is necessary for the synthesis of myelin and neurotransmitters. Iron is needed for conversion of 5-HT, 5 hydroxytroptamine, to serotonin. [109] This may be helpful if you are sluggish in the morning.

Iron metabolism

1. Energy. Iron is needed for cytchromes in mitochondria or simply put, "no iron no ATP". Iron is needed for metabolism of lysine to carnitine.
2. Neurotransmitters. Iron is needed for serotonin and melatonin synthesis.
3. Hormones. Iron aids steroid synthesis.
4. Hemoglobin. Iron is a very important part of red blood cells.
5. Vitamin C.
Caution: excess iron can damage tissue from oxidation.[110] This has to do with the Fenton reaction.
A decrease in stomach acidity can decrease iron absorption.[111] Stomach acidity may be decreased in people with this disease. This would help to explain the low iron levels on my blood tests.

---

[109] Merck Manual, Fifteenth Edition, 1987, page 942
[110] http://ncbI.nlm.nih.gov.entrez/iron
[111] http://lpi.oregonstate.edu/infocenter/minerals/iron/index.html

CHAPTER 24

Sexual Promiscuity

Too hot, gotta trot

Sexual arousal probably occurs more frequently and more easily with people that have this disease. This may be due to increased nitric oxide production or, perhaps, because of nitrogen metabolism is affected. I have not investigated this aspect to any significant degree. This affect on nitrogen metabolism may help explain some of the promiscuous behavior exhibited by people with this disease. *I was promiscuous prior to marriage.*

Nitrogen is excreted excessively in metabolic acidosis. Acidosis can be improved by growth hormone. Nitrogen is a component or urea and ammonia. Both compounds are vitally involved in kidney function. Ammonia is a buffer. **Excessive levels of ammonia are neurotoxic. Glutamate metabolism and other pathways produce ammonia. Excessively high glutamate levels have been associated with attention deficit disorder. Note that sexual stimulation involves nitric oxide. This is the molecule that is associated with the activity of Viagra. This may explain some of the sexual behavior of bipolar people.**

The question then becomes, "Are children with Attention Deficit Disorder more sexually promiscuous?"

The main source nitrogen is the removal of ammonia (NH3) from the amino acid glutamine, which is turned into glutamate. The enzyme glutaminase, abundantly present in renal tubular cells, catalyses the reaction. The glutamate in turn can give up another ammonia molecule, to form alpha-ketoglutarate. Ever cunning, the kidney then can metabolize the alpha-ketoglutarate, using two hydrogen ions in the process! All in all, this is a smart way of getting rid of ammonia, and removing hydrogen ions. (Nitrous oxide is laughing gas). Note that the glutamate comes mainly from the liver, which thus participates indirectly in acid-base balance. Note that for the reaction:

$NH_3 + H^+ <==> NH_4^+$

the pK' is 9.0, in other words, only at a pH of 9.0 will equal concentrations of ammonia and ammonium be present at equilibrium. The lower the pH (more acidic, more ammonium ion), the higher the concentration of ammonium ion that is relative to that of ammonia. This is a wonderful mechanism for concentrating ammonium ion in the urine—the renal cells make ammonia which diffuses into the urine, hydrogen ions in the urine bind the ammonia to make ammonium, and more ammonia can therefore diffuse passively across the renal cells into the urine, to be snapped up in turn![112]

---

[112] http://www.anaesthetist.com/icu/elec/nagacid/htm

SECTION 3

PHYSIOLOGY

CHAPTER 25

The Bile System and Mineral Losses

How are the trace elements being lost?

I noticed a very slight jaundice color to my sons skin when he was getting sick. I now know why. It was not overtly yellow, but just a small change in tint. I occasionally have a mild spasm in the area where my gall bladder would be located. I don't know if this is abnormal or not because it is normal to me.

Bile is a complex fluid containing water, electrolytes and a battery of organic molecules including bile acids, cholesterol, phospholipids and bilirubin that flows through the biliary tract into the small intestine.[113]

The rate-limiting enzyme for bile acid synthesis is 7 alpha hydroxylase.[114] This enzyme requires a niacin analog to perform this reaction. Note that niacin deficiency may cause grasping reflex. I experience this. If bile secretion is down regulated, then there may be an effect on metals that are excreted via the biliary system. The expectation would be a higher concentration of these ions in organ tissue or, perhaps, there may be a system that down-regulates absorption. Again, note this is a rate-limited reaction, which requires a metal cofactor. I believe this is possibly the reason my bilirubin level result was low. Note that many hydroxylase enzymes are either produced or secreted via bile salts.

---

113 http://arbl.cvmbs.colostate.edu/hbooks/pathphys/digestion/liver/bile.html
114 Harrison's Principles of Internal Medicine, 10th edition, page 1823.

Bile acids perform four physiologically significant functions:
- 1. Their synthesis and subsequent excretion in the feces represent the only significant mechanism for the elimination of excess cholesterol.
- 2. Bile acids and phospholipids solubilize cholesterol in the bile, thereby preventing the precipitation of cholesterol in the gallbladder.
- 3. They facilitate the digestion of dietary triacylglycerols by acting as emulsifying agents that render fats accessible to pancreatic lipases.
- 4. They facilitate the intestinal absorption of **fat-soluble vitamins.**[115]

The gall bladder stores and concentrates bile during the fasting state.[116]

Secretin is secreted in response to acid in the duodenum. Its effect on the biliary system is very similar to what was seen in the pancreas—it simulates biliary duct cells to secrete bicarbonate and water, which expands the volume of bile and increases its flow out into the intestine.[117] Chewing gum may stimulate secretin production. I have noticed that when I chew gum, I do so with vigor.

There seems to be a detrimental effect on fat-soluble vitamins in this disease. Notice the night blindness associated with a deficiency in the fat-soluble vitamin A. Again, the fat-soluble vitamin D is affected. A vitamin K defect, which may be caused by manganese deficiency, may be the reason for increased bleeding times.

Although I do not believe that achlorhydria presents itself prominently in this disease; I do believe hypochlorhydria does. Achlorhydria is defined as failure of the intragastric pH to fall to less than 4.0 under maximal stimulation (with pentagastrin). It may develop as a result of several conditions and may or may not be reversible. Acid production is not possible once the acid-producing gastric mucosa has been destroyed

This is an autoimmune gastritis that involves the fundic glands. In this condition, fundic histology is characterized by severe gland atrophy. **Ninety percent of patients have antibodies directed against the H^+/K^+-ATPase pump.** In these patients, achlorhydria leads to pronounced hypergastrinemia (>1000 pg/mL) with subsequent hyperplasia of gastric enterochromaffinlike cells. Gastric carcinoid tumors develop in 3-5% of patients. Pernicious anemia also

---

[115] http://web.indstate.edu/thcme/mwking/cholesterol.html#bile
[116] http://arbl.cvmbs.colostate.edu/hbooks/pathphys/digestion/liver/bile.html
[117] http://arbl.cvmbs.colostate.edu/hbooks/pathphys/digestion/liver/bile.ht

leads to vitamin B-12 malabsorption, in which the absence of intrinsic factor produced by the stomach mucosa and its cellular source leads to the vitamin B-12 deficiency. **Autoimmune thyroid disease is commonly observed in association with autoimmune gastritis**[118] These early experiments identified three separable routes for chloride secretion: an active transport component, an ion-exchange component, and a **passive ionic diffusion component** [119] I believe passive diffusion may play a role in hyperchloremic acidosis.

Alkaline phosphatase inhibits secretin-stimulated bile flow and bicarbonate secretion.[120] (Please note usually low levels of alkaline phosphatase in my blood work). Secretin is a 27-amino acid neuroendocrine peptide. It is synthesized by specific endocrine cells, S cells, located mainly in the mucosa of the duodenum and proximal jejunum. Secretin regulates the physiological functions of many organs including the brain (e.g., activation of **tyrosine hydroxylase activity**) pancreas, intestine, and liver. Secretin stimulates the gastric secretion of pepsin and inhibits the secretion of gastric acid and food-stimulated gastrin from G cells in the gastric antrum. Furthermore, secretin affects the motility of the small intestine, decreases lower esophageal sphincter pressure, relaxes the sphincter of Oddi, and inhibits postprandial emptying. Secretin.increases heart rate and causes dilatation of peripheral blood vessels.[121]

The liver and bile system are involved with several very important functions like:

(1) **metabolic functions**, such as the **maintenance of glucose (blood sugar) levels**
(2) **synthetic functions**, such as the **synthesis of serum proteins** such as albumin, blood clotting (coagulation) factors, and complement (a mediator of inflammatory responses)
(3) **storage functions**, such as the **storage of sugar (glycogen), fat (triglycerides), iron, copper, and fat-soluble vitamins (A, D, E, and K)**. (4) Catabolic functions, such as the detoxification of drugs.[122]

Several other metabolic reactions require vitamin C as a cofactor. These include the catabolism of tyrosine and the synthesis of epinephrine from tyrosine and the synthesis of the bile acids.[123]

---

[118] http://author.emedicine.com/MED/topic18.htm
[119] http://ajpgi.physiology.org/cgi/content/full/283/5/G1147
[120] http://ajpgi.physiology.org/cgi/content/full/281/3/G612/T1
[121] http://ajpgi.physiology.org/cgi/content/full/281/3/G612
[122] http://pathology2.jhu.edu/bileduct/anatphys.cfm
[123] http://www.indstate.edu/thcme/mwking/vitamins.html

Liver disease decreases storage capacity, transport, and activation of many nutrients. *Iron, folate, vitamin B_{12}, riboflavin, niacin, vitamin B_6 stores may be substantially depleted.* Nutrient transport is impaired by decreased hepatic synthesis of albumin, retinol-binding protein, ceruloplasmin, transferrin, and lipoproteins. Hypoalbuminemia promotes fluid retention and increases potential for neurotoxic effects of tryptophan and bilirubin. Vitamin D activation is inhibited in the presence of normal renal function because the first step occurs in the liver. Urea synthesis is impaired which promotes the accumulation of ammonia and increases risk of encephalopathy. *Hypoglycemia may be present in acute liver disease, which is replaced with insulin resistance in chronic liver disease.* Protein and fluid restriction are key nutritional adjustments to liver disease that need to be made. *Anorexia* is a common feature.[124]

Hypoglycemia, hypoproteinemia, reduced fat stores, anemia, copper pathway failure, vitamin D failure, vitamin K failure, and night blindness associated with vitamin A are all problems I have noticed. Note that these are subclinical problems. They are produced not from failure, but from inefficiency.

Vitamin C is involved with the immune system. Vitamin C is needed for white cell function. **Vitamin C is needed also for energy. It is needed for conversion of lysine to carnitine. Carnitine is necessary as muscle fuel.** Vitamin C is needed for serotonin and melatonin production as well as dopamine and NE production. Vitamin C deficiency may result in sleep disturbances and possibly depression. Vitamin C is needed to produce cortisol and adrenalin. Vitamin C acts as an antioxidant and metal scavenger. Vitamin C is involved in tissue repair and vitamin C deficiency may result in bruises and bleeding gums. High levels of copper renders vitamin C useless. **Vitamin C actions stimulate hydroxylase.**[125]

Vitamin C is involved in collagen, bone and teeth formation. Vitamin C is involved in wound healing and burn recovery. Vitamin C is involved in cellular redox reactions. Vitamin C protects folic acid reductase. Vitamin C helps to release folic acid from food. Vitamin C aids iron absorption. Cold or heat stress increases vitamin C excretion. (This may in some way explain heat sensitivity in bipolar people). *Bleeding gums and hyperkeratotic hair follicles are physical signs of deficiency.* (I have experienced this). Norepinephrine is synthe-

---

[124] www.nums.nwu.edu/nutrition/tools-resources/sbm-files/
SBM-NutrDiseaseTrauma.doc

[125] http://www.nutritionreviewservice.com.au/recap.PDF

sized in the adrenal gland and requires vitamin C. Vitamin C helps to metabolize cholesterol to bile acids.[126] Vitamin C requires copper and iron as cofactors.[127] The most important reaction requiring ascorbate as a cofactor is the *hydroxylation* of proline residues in collagen.[128]

It appears, biochemically speaking, that vitamin C and vitamin B6 act hand in hand in the hydroxylation and decarboxylation process. I believe using supplement of these and their cofactors are warranted in this disease.

[126] Merck Manual, Fifteenth Edition, 1987, page 939

[127] http://www.Expasy (Roche Biochemical Pathway)

[128] http://www.indstate.edu/thcme/mwking/vitamins.html

CHAPTER 26

Stomach Acid Secretion, Belching, and Flatulence

Malabsorption, starving in the midst of plenty

Prior to my hospitalization in 1991, I was belching several times an hour. It wasn't painful, just annoying. I did not have any other symptoms that were strong enough to require my seeking medical attention. Most of the time, my symptoms could be controlled with an over-the-counter antacid like Zantac.

I had gas daily. I may sound strange, but there are different smells of "poots". There is your normal methane gas. There is also chlorine, phosphorous, and sulfur "poots". I believe each type tells something about what is happening physiologically. Phosphorus gas smells like matches and sulfur gas smells like sulfur. Chlorine gas I believe is odorless as is carbon dioxide. I believe in states of hyperchloremia excess chloride ion is converted to chlorine gas which is expelled through a GI orifice. *I am sure my friends are glad to know I no longer experience any significant amount of belching or flatulence.*

The hydrogen ion concentration in parietal cell secretions is roughly 3 million fold higher than in blood, and chloride is secreted against both a concentration and electric gradient. Thus, the ability of the partietal cell to secrete acid is dependent on active transport.

The key player in acid secretion is a H+/K+ ATPase or "proton pump" located in the cannalicular membrane. This ATPase is **magnesium-dependent,** and not inhibitable by ouabain. The current model for explaining acid secretion is as follows:

- Hydrogen ions are generated within the parietal cell from dissociation of water. The hydroxyl ions formed in this process rapidly combine with carbon dioxide to form bicarbonate ion, a reaction cataylzed by **carbonic anhydrase.**

- Bicarbonate is transported out of the basolateral membrane in exchange for chloride. The outflow of bicarbonate into blood results in a slight elevation of blood pH known as the "alkaline tide". This process serves to maintain intracellular pH in the parietal cell.
- Chloride and **potassium** ions are transported into the lumen of the cannaliculus by conductance channels, and such is necessary for secretion of acid.
- Hydrogen ion is pumped out of the cell, into the lumen, in exchange for potassium through the action of the proton pump; potassium is thus effectively recycled.
- Accumulation of osmotically-active hydrogen ion in the cannaliculus generates an osmotic gradient across the membrane that results in outward diffusion of water—the resulting gastric juice is 155 mM HCl and 15 mM KCl with a small amount of NaCl. [129]

(With possible deficiencies in potassium, magnesium and carbonic anhydrase, hypochlorhydria would be expected producing a mild malabsorption syndrome.)

Researchers have found a selective metal transporter called DMTI in the bile. **All the metals transported by DMT1 (Fe^{2+}, Zn^{2+}, Mn^{2+}, Co^{2+}, Cd^{2+}, Cu^{2+}, Ni^{2+}, and Pb^{2+}) readily form coordination complexes in aqueous solution, with different preferences for coordinating atoms.** Coordination would support the pH findings: if the proton current functioned as an electrochemical gradient, increasing the transmembrane gradient (lower extracellular pH) would increase uptake, as occurs in the proton-driven transport of dipolar amino acids across intestinal epithelia.[130]

---

[129] http://www.vivo.colostate.edu/hbooks/pathphys/digestion/stomach/parietal.html
[130] http://ajpgi.physiology.org/cgi/content/full/279/6/G1265

CHAPTER 27

Parathyroid Endocrinology

What is the cause of mania?

Hypomania is an exhilarating feeling. You literally feel "on top of the world". Some clinicians believe this is the reason many bipolar patients quit taking their medicine. It is during these periods of hypomania that bipolar artists and writers have produced many of our greatest works of art and literature. In a hypomanic state I was everyone's friend, jovial and with a ribald sense of humor.

I found a common description of bipolar disease at bipolarworld.net. Mania on the other hand takes on the reins of irrationality. The poet Robert Lowell described his mania as "pathological enthusiasm".

Bipolar I Disorder brings with it:

1. Changes in mood for a distinct period of time—feeling happy, optimistic, euphoric, irritable
2. Changes in thinking—thoughts speeding through one's brain, unrealistic self confidence, difficulty concentrating, grandiose plans, delusions, hallucinations
3. Changes in behavior—increased activity or socializing, immersion in plans or projects, talking very rapidly and excessively, excessive spending, impaired judgment, impulsive sexual involvement
4. Changes in physical condition—less need for sleep, increased energy, fewer health complaints. Nine out of ten people with Bipolar I Disorder also experience depression including depressed mood, loss of interest in activities, feelings of worthlessness and hopelessness, lack of appetite, sleep difficulties, lack of energy and thoughts of suicide.

Manic Behavior you might observe:

Generally an episode seems to begin overnight with a sudden and pleasant switch of mood to one of well-being, lightening, happiness and positive energy. At this stage (known as mild mania or hypomania) the individual is able to function quite well, and this mood may persist at this level for a long period of time without becoming more severe. In other cases it intensifies day by day into true mania. This is the state I will discuss here.

- Out of control of emotions and behavior…Very distressed
- Normally amiable people may become increasingly angry, impulsive, emotional or irritable
- Intense *euphoria* that nothing can disturb, but if their plans are foiled they may become irritable or uncontrollably furious
- Some may become hostile
- A few manics may become *paranoid or violent* and assault others verbally or physically
- Very *rapid speech*, incessant and usually in a loud voice
- Answer questions at great length and continue talking when others speak
- Speech may be riddled with jokes, puns, or irrelevant witticisms
- Acting in *theatrical* roles and ways
- Offer money or advice to passing strangers
- Unable to sleep or sit still…often going for days with 2 or3 hrs sleep and not feeling tired
- *Socially frenetic*…throwing parties, going to bars
- Throw aside normal inhibitions and become sexually hyperactive or promiscuous
- Due to impaired judgment very *poor decision making* skills. Overspending, over commitment, quitting jobs, etc.

In persons with extreme mania you may see some of the following:

- Thinking completely *illogical*
- Speech uncontrollable and sometimes *incoherent*
- *Unable to distinguish between "real" and "not real"*
- *Delusions, paranoia, hallucinations*
- Catatonia possible[131]

---

[131] http://www.bipolarworld.net/Diagnosis/Diagnosis/mania.html

I believe it is very important to understand that only one kidney may be affected. I have right kidney awareness. I do not call it pain. If as I theorize that only one kidney is affected then treating this disease may be more difficult. Imagine the brain trying to figure out was is going on when it gets signals from one that says everything is okay and the other kidney is giving different signals. The brain is thinking, "How can I compensate?" If you can imagine an old movie serial where two guys are on a train fighting for control of the throttle; one is pushing, the other is pulling. The speed of the ride is very erratic. Imagine the guy pushing manages to throw off the pulling guy. The pushing guy then manages to go full throttle. In human terms we call this mania. However, the pulling guy climbs back aboard and the fight over the throttle continues. So the high rate of speed lasts only a short time. Imagine the guy tossing the coal into the engine does not know the fight is happening, but he senses the change of speed and tosses in even more coal in hope to speed up the train. This only makes the engine get so hot it might explode. If this happens the train wrecks. In human terms we call this psychosis.

We shall learn a great deal more about these glands in the following paragraphs. The PARATHYROIDS, 4 tiny glands embedded in the thyroid gland, produces parathormone, which regulates calcium and phosphate metabolism.[132]

It was now August, about 4 months after my son's hospitalization. I had contacted an old friend from my college days who was now a professor of pharmacy and I related to her my feelings about lithium. Lithium carbonate is the drug of choice in bipolar disease. Lithium is another alkali. I had read somewhere that "lithium only worked for bipolar disease if it was in the carbonate form." I felt that the obvious and overlooked thing is that it was the carbonate, not the lithium, which was critical. This hypothesis intrigued her and it was a discovery in the Merck Manual that helped propel research. The important question was "If this is a kidney disease then what causes the mood swings?" I found that answer in Merck. There is a reference to **"secondary hypoparathyroidism and pseudohyperparathyroidism"** coexisting in cases of nephrogenic diabetes insipidus, also known as distal renal tubular acidosis, diagnosis. According to Merck, "In some patients with hypoparathyroidism and pseudohyperparathyroidism, subnormal formation of 1,25-DHCC may contribute to the relative refractoriness of hypocalcemia to correction by vitamin D." [133] The bipolar theory suggests that

---

[132] http://www.duke.edu/~djs3/bio/
[133] Merck Manual, Fifteenth edition, 1987, page 971.

hypomania and mania occurs during the periods of pseudohyperparathyroidism when phosphate ion deficiency stimulates direct reabsorption of phosphate ion. This increase in circulating phosphate would stimulate vitamin activity, particularly thiamine and pyridoxine because they are phosphate salts. In other words, thiamine and pyridoxine require adequate levels of phosphate to do their work. This reabsorptive phase is brief, which would explain the short timespan of hypo mania. **The bipolar theory suggests that bipolar patients spend a significant amount of time as a hypo parathyroid person due to 1,25 DHCC failure. It is the direct stimulation for phosphate reabsorption that produces the mood swing.** My theory suggests that not only does the phosphate correct acidosis temporarily, but the additional phosphate is incorporated quickly forming restoring ATP levels. The normalized ATP levels gives the bipolar person that burst of energy that is referred to as hypo mania).

Maintaining normal blood calcium and phosphorus concentrations is managed through the concerted action of three hormones that control fluxes of calcium in and out of blood and extracellular fluid:

Parathyroid hormone serves to increase blood concentrations of calcium. Mechanistically, parathyroid hormone preserves blood calcium by several major effects:

- Stimulates production of the biologically-active form of vitamin D within the kidney.
- Facilitates mobilization of calcium and phosphate from bone. To prevent detrimental increases in phosphate, **parathyroid hormone also has a potent effect on the kidney to eliminate phosphate (phosphaturic effect).**
- Maximizes tubular reabsorption of calcium within the kidney. This activity results in minimal losses of calcium in urine.

Vitamin D acts also to increase blood concentrations of calcium. It is generated through the activity of parathyroid hormone within the kidney. Far and away the most important effect of vitamin D is to facilitate absorption of calcium from the small intestine. In concert with parathyroid hormone, vitamin D also enhances fluxes of calcium out of bone.

Calcitonin is a hormone that functions to reduce blood calcium levels. It is secreted in response to hypercalcemia and has at least two effects:

- Suppression of renal tubular reabsorption of calcium. In other words, calcitonin enhances excretion of calcium into urine.
- Inhibition of bone resorption, which would minimize fluxes of calcium from bone into blood.

Although calcitonin has significant calcium-lowing effects in some species, it appears to have a minimal influence on blood calcium levels in humans.[134]

Secondary hyperparathyroidism occurs when the parathyroid gland is chronically stimulated to release parathyroid hormone. This can be caused by malabsorption syndromes, chronic renal failure and "rickets." Laboratory results include elevated serum chloride levels, decreased serum phosphate levels, decreased serum carbon dioxide, hyperchloremic metabolic acidosis, and increase in urine cyclic adenosine monophosphate (cAMP). [135]

The Bipolar Parathyroid Gland

Hypoparathyroidism is the state of decreased secretion or activity of parathyroid hormone (PTH). **This leads to decreased blood levels of calcium (hypocalcemia) and increased levels of blood phosphorus (hyperphosphatemia).**[136] (The body is compensating for phosphate losses). The element magnesium is closely related to the action of calcium in the body. When magnesium levels are too low, calcium levels may also fall. It appears that magnesium is important for parathyroid cells to make PTH normally. Once recognized, this is usually very easy to fix. Chronic alcoholism is a frequent cause of low calcium and magnesium levels.[137]

The major regulatory signal for PTH secretion is serum calcium (Table 17) (11). **Serum calcium inversely affects PTH secretion,** with the steep portion of the sigmoidal response curve corresponding to the normal range of both. An increase in ionized calcium inhibits PTH secretion by increasing intracellular calcium through the release of calcium from intracellular stores and the influx of extracellular calcium through cell membranes and channels. This mechanism differs from most cells, where secretion of their product is stimulated by increased calcium. Intracellular magnesium may serve this secretory function in the parathyroids in that hypermagnesemia can inhibit PTH secretion and hypomagnesemia can stimulate PTH secretion. However, prolonged depletion of magnesium will inhibit PTH biosynthesis and secretion, as it will the function of many cells. Hypomagnesemia also attenuates the biological effect of PTH.[138]

---

[134] http://arbl.cvmbs.colostate.edu/hbooks/pathphys/endocrine/thyroid/
calcium.html

[135] http://www.emedicine.com/emerg/topic265.htm

[136] http://endocrineweb.com/0_old/hypopara.html

[137] http://endocrineweb.com/0_old/hypopara.html

[138] http://www.endotext.com/parathyroid/parathyroid2/parathyroidframe2.htm

Parathyroid hormone actions include (1) rapid mobilization of calcium and phosphate from bone and long term acceleration of bone resorption (2) increased renal tubular reabsorption of calcium, (3) increased intestinal aborption via vitamin D, (4) decrease renal tubular reabsorption of phosphate. **Decreased levels of alkaline phosphatases signify hypoparathyroidism and/or hypophosphatemia.**[139]*

About 40% of free Calcium is protein bound in the blood. The other 60% of free Calcium is unilateral and includes ionized calcium plus calcium complexed with phosphate and citrate. Acidosis is associated with decreased protein binding (note that bipolar patient's have lower than normal levels of protein) and increased ionized calcium. These pH changes occur independently of any change in total blood calcium concentration. Parathyroid hormone and vitamin D are principal regulators of calcium and phosphate. Parathyroid hormone causes increased active vitamin D. Decreased vitamin D causes decreased parathyroid action.

The net effects of PTH activity are an increase in serum calcium and a decrease in serum phosphate. PTH acts directly upon bone to stimulate bone resorption and cause calcium and phosphate release. PTH acts directly upon the kidney to decrease calcium clearance and to inhibit phosphate reabsorption. By stimulating renal 1 alpha hydroxylase activity, PTH increase serum concentrations of 1,25 dihydroxyvitamin D, the active form of vitamin D and, thus, indirectly stimulates calcium and phosphate absorption by the gut through the actions of vitamin D. The phosphaturic effect of PTH offsets the increases of serum phosphate driven by increased bone resorption and GI absorption. Hypoparathyroidism results in loss of both the direct and indirect effects of PTH on bone, the kidney, and the gut. Calcium and phosphate release from bone is impaired, calcium absorption from the gut is limited, calciuria develops despite hypocalcemia, and retention of phosphate from the urine causes increased plasma phosphate levels.[140] *A person with bipolar disease has probably experienced both sets of symptoms, i.e., hyperparathyroidism and hypoparathyroidism.*

In the kidney, PTH increases the reabsorption of calcium, predominantly in the distal convoluted tubule, and inhibits the reabsorption of phosphate in

---

[139] Merck Manual, Fifteenth Edition, 1987, page 843
[140] http://emedicine.com/ped/topic1125.htm

the renal proximal tubule, causing hypercalcemia and hypophosphatemia. PTH also inhibits NA+?H+ antiporter activity and bicarbonate reabsorption, causing a mild hyperchloremic metabolic acidosis.[141]

The elevated PTH and hypercalcemia levels found in this condition can differentiate hyperparathyroidism easily. Renal leak hypercalciuria has secondary hyperparathyroidism but no hypercalcemia. Renal phosphate leak shows elevated urinary phosphate and reduced serum phosphate, as well as elevated vitamin D blood levels. [142]

Major sites of regulation of phosphate excretion are the early proximal renal tubule and the distal convoluted tubule. In the proximal tubule, phosphate reabsorption by type II sodium-phosphate cotransporters is regulated by dietary phosphate, PTH, and vitamin D.

High dietary phosphate intake and elevated PTH levels decrease proximal renal tubule phosphate absorption, thus enhancing renal excretion. Conversely, low dietary phosphate intake, low PTH levels, and high vitamin D levels enhance renal proximal tubule phosphate absorption.

To some extent, phosphate regulates its own regulators. High phosphate concentrations in the blood down-regulate the expression of some phosphate transporters, decrease vitamin D production, and increase PTH secretion by the parathyroid gland. Distal tubule phosphate handling is less well understood. PTH increases phosphate reabsorption in the distal tubule, but the mechanisms by which this occurs are unknown. Renal phosphate excretion can also be increased by the administration of loop diuretics.[143]

Inadequate phosphate intake alone is an uncommon cause of hypophosphatemia.[144] Increased excretion of phosphate is a more common mechanism for the development of hypophosphatemia. The most common cause of increased renal phosphate excretion is hyperparathyroidism due to the ability of PTH to inhibit proximal renal tubule phosphate transport.[145] Vitamin D deficiency not only impairs intestinal absorption, but also decreases renal absorption of phosphate.[146]

Glucocorticoids induce phosphaturia, and decreased tubular reabsorption of phosphate has been reported 254 208. These effects can be attributed in large part

---

[141] http://www.endotext.com/parathyroid/parathyroid2/parathyroidframe2.htm

[142] http://author.emedicine.com/MED/topic1069.htm

[143] http://www.emedicine.com/med/topic1135.htm

[144] http://www.emedicine.com/med/topic1135.htm

[145] http://www.emedicine.com/med/topic1135.htm

[146] http://www.emedicine.com/med/topic1135.htm

to secondary hyperparathyroidism; however, glucocorticoids have also direct effects on the kidney.[147] Cortisol, a glucocorticoid, is secreted normally twice a day. The times are usually 4 a.m. and 2 p.m. These are also periods of significant sleep. If you experience significant "afternoon swoon" your phosphate levels are probably low.

The active form of vitamin D enhances calcium transport (absorption) and enhances phosphate transport (absorption). [148] Urinary calcium excretion is increased by high protein intake.[149] *See the blood test.

---

[147] http://www.endotext.com/adrenal/adrenal7/adrenalframe7.htm
[148] Merck Manual, Fifteenth Edition, 1987, page 1960
[149] Harrison's Principles of Internal Medicine, 10th Edition, page 1923

CHAPTER 28

Vitamin D and Energy Loss

Why am I so tired?

Here I made a critical mistake in treatment, which ultimately led me to the final discovery. Vitamin D has been described as a cross between a hormone and a vitamin. The synthesis of vitamin D begins in the skin through the stimulation of special cells that are sensitive to sunlight. It is important to remember that the parathyroid and vitamin D are inherently integrated. I tried to simplify the regimen by using a product called Boost. Boost is an excellent product with virtually all the nutrients, minerals and vitamins, in a palatable liquid form. We began using this regularly and initially everything seemed to be working fine. My son, however, was steadily getting worse and I could not explain this.

Distal Renal Tubular Acidosis as defined by Harrison's is the failure of bicarbonate to be reabsorbed and phosphate is excreted normally by the distal tubule in the kidney causing acidosis due to excessive chlorine reabsorption. I kept researching phosphate reabsorption. I made the connection to calcium since they are usually appear as "pairs" in the body. In other words, you find one and the other is usually not too far behind. The same can be said for sodium and chloride. I began looking at calcium reabsorption in the distal tubule. I found our old friend, vitamin D. However, there are many forms of vitamin D. The active form of vitamin D is hydroxylated in the distal renal tubule to form 1,25 dihydroxy vitamin D3. The active form of vitamin D enhances calcium transport (absorption) and enhances phosphate transport (absorption). [150] Urinary calcium excretion is increased by high protein intake.[151]

Note that phosphate is actively reabsorbed via sodium pump in the upper portion of the descending limb. This pump is sensitive to parathyroid hormone. In an attempt to maintain calcium levels the body requests intake of

---

[150] Merck Manual, Fifteenth Edition, 1987, page 1960
[151] Harrison's Principles of Internal Medicine, 10th Edition, page 1923

more calcium. The major source for calcium nutrition is obtained by drinking milk. Everyone is probably saying, "Well, this a good thing." There is a problem there however. Milk is now fortified with vitamin D. A person with bipolar disease who consumes extremely large quantities of milk will from time to time experience vitamin D toxicity. This toxicity produces its own set of problems.

I had always been a big milk drinker. My Dad used to purchase ten gallons of milk for us when I was a child. I was the biggest consumer in this household. I was also the moodiest. I knew that this craving for milk must mean there was a calcium deficiency somehow. I drank more than enough milk. The question was "Why am I not absorbing the calcium?" Reabsorbing in this case. I investigated milks contents, (1) calcium, primarily (2) phosphate, a reasonably amount, but not as high as I had expected and (3) vitamin D, about 25 i.u. units per cup. Note that a cup is one-half glassful. The upper limit for an adult is for vitamin D is 200 i.u. Make note that your body makes vitamin D. It does not have to come from extraneous sources if you get enough sunshine. The sun actually activates melatonin in the skin to produce this vitamin. Now I calculated that if I drank 4 glasses of milk per day (the equivalent of 8 cupfuls), which is not an unusual amount for me, that would be 200 i.u.! I used to drink milk like most people drink water. If I ate anything with significant amounts of vitamin D in addition or if I received considerable UV sun exposure I was in the toxic range. I looked up Vitamin D toxicity in Merck Manual. I found some startling information.

Vitamin D, parathyroid hormone and insulin are all related compounds. Symptoms of hyperparathyroidism coincide with vitamin D toxicity. Renal symptoms include thirst, frequent drinking, and frequent urination. These symptoms also correspond to those for the disease diabetes insipidous. Toxic vitamin D gastro-intestinal symptoms include abdominal distress, constipation, vomiting, anorexia, and weight loss. Mental symptoms include anxiety, depression, psychosis, apathy, and fatigue. Physical symptoms are fatigue, neurophysciatric illness, and decreased mental alertness and muscle pain. Pancreatitis and peptic ulcer disease may occur. Cardiovascular signs include hypertension and congestive heart failure.

Toxic levels of vitamin D symptoms include anorexia, nausea, and vomiting, followed by frequent urination, frequent thirst and water intake, weakness, nervousness, and pruritis. I have had all of those symptoms at some time or another throughout my lifetime. Vitamin D toxicity occurs commonly during treatment of hypoparathyroidism. [152] *My theory suggests that the vitamin D precursors in high levels produce these side effects.*

---

[152] Merck Manual, Fifteenth Edition, 1987, page 974.

I learned about the macula densa, a portion of the kidney where vitamin D is activated. I knew from my pharmacy career that an activated vitamin D (calcitriol) supplement existed. At my August appointment last year I was unable to convince my psychiatrist of the need for calcitriol. I kept looking at the system. I typed into the computer on my Dad's birthday, he had passed away only a year before, the word: hydroxylase. I followed down to a site on emedicine that described 1 alpha hydroxylase. It stated that **1 alpha hydroxylase** is responsible for the conversion of vitamin D3 to 1,25 DHCC or calcitriol. Emedicine also stated that the parathyroid could be affected to synthesize more 1 alpha hydroxylase by calcium loading. [153] I purchased a bottle of Tum's Extra Strength. I ate 6 tablets that night. My voice has always been sensitive to this disease. Sometimes my voice was high and raspy and, however, there were times when I felt well when my voice would be deep and full. I believed if this worked my voice would be low. The next morning I awoke to a deep voice. Hurray! This was a breakthrough. My kidneys were now producing enough 1,25 DHCC to stimulate absorption of enough phosphate from the gut.

---

[153] http://arbl.cvmbs.colostate.edu/hbooks/pathphys/endocrine/
thryoid/calcium.html

Calcium-Loading Test Interpretation Guide

Criteria	Absorptive Type I Vitamin D– Dependent, Classic Type	Absorptive Type I Vitamin D– Dependent, Variant Type	Absorptive Type II Dietary Calcium Responsive	Absorptive Type III (Renal Phosphate Leak)	Renal Calcium Leak
Urinary calcium on regular diet[†]	High	High	High	High	High
Urinary calcium on low-calcium diet[‡]	High	High	NL	High	High
Urinary calcium fasting[§]	NL	High	NL	High	High
Urinary calcium after 1-g calcium load[‖]	High	High	NL	High	High
Serum PO_4 fasting	NL	NL	NL	Low	NL or high
Serum calcium fasting	NL	NL or high	NL	NL or high	NL or low
Serum PTH	NL or low	NL or low	NL	Low	High
Serum PTH after 1-g calcium load	NL or low	NL or low**	NL	Low	**High**
Serum vitamin D-3 (calcitriol)	NL	High	NL	High	High
Fasting normocalciuria while on ketoconazol	No	Yes	No	Yes	No
Bone calcium	NL	NL or low	NL	NL or low	Low

*Resorptive means hyperparathyroidism.

†Regular diet is unrestricted calcium and sodium intake. Normal upper limit calciuria is <4 mg/kg body weight per day.

‡Low-calcium diet is 400 mg calcium and 100 mEq of sodium per day. Normal upper limit calciuria is <200 mg/d.

§Fasting is a 12 hour fast. Normal upper limit is <0.11 mg calcium/mg creatinine.

[II]After 1-g calcium load, normal upper limit is <0.20 mg calcium/mg creatinine.[154]

**(Lower PTH means higher serum phosphate, calcium-loading causing a decrease in PTH which causes increased phosphate reabsorption.)

Vitamin C is involved in hydroxylase synthesis. The amino acids lysine and proline affected in particular. Copper and vitamin C are involved with lysine hydroxylation in collagen synthesis. **Vitamin C and copper are involved with dopamine beta hydroxylase.**[155] I thought that by supplementing vitamin C, iron, and copper to my diet maybe the production of 1,25 DHCC will increased as well. Naturally produced vitamin D from sun synthesis may be the best source of vitamin D. However, do not overdo any other of these suggestions because they all have toxicities. Listen to your body. My theory states that it is important to avoid excess provitamin D because of side effects. My theory also states that it is important to stimulate 1 alpha hydroxylase by two methods, (1) calcium loading and (2) vitamin C and iron/copper supplementation. Twenty minutes of sunshine three times a week appears to provide enough vitamin D naturally.

Several hormones effect phosphate reabsorption by the kidney. Among these parathyroid hormone, calcitonin, glucocorticoids and phosphate loading inhibit renal phosphate reclamation. In contrast, growth hormone, insulin, thyroid hormone, 1,25DHCC, and phosphate deprivation (depletion) stimulate renal phosphate reabsorption. The common target for this hormonal regulation is the renal proximal tubular cell.[156] I understand from this statement that a body trying to increase phosphate levels may secrete more growth hormone and grow taller. Perhaps, that is what happened to me. The affect the insulin has on phosphate reabsorption may help explain the "sweet tooth." By eating sweets insulin levels would become dramatically elevated, which would allow more phosphate reabsorption.

---

154 http://author.emedicine.com/MED/topic1069.htm
155 http://www.aamm.unm.edu/vitamin cofactors
156 http://www.endotext.org/parathyroid/parathryoid10/parathyroid10.htm

SECTION 4

STRESS, DRUGS,
AND SUICIDE

CHAPTER 29

Stress and Psychosis

"Uneasy lies the head that wears a crown."

My younger brother used to love to slowly come to me from behind and scare me out of my wits. I believe this heightened vigilance is due to an over-production of cortisol or at least an increased sensitivity to cortisol.

The ADRENAL glands, which sit on top of each kidney, produces 2 hormones: adrenaline that is responsible for your "flight or fight" response; and cortisol, that plays a role in regulating glucose level in the blood.[157]

All of this explained bipolar disease, but it did not adequately explain why psychosis occurs in some and not in others. I began researching the role of stress. I found that excess chloride ion directly affected the sensitivity of the adrenal glands and that the increased production of cortisol releasing factor or CRF caused an increased sensitivity of this system. In other words, an untreated person with bipolar disease begins the day with a higher stress level than the normal person. So once additional stress is added the system over-loads. **Considering that the minerals of a bipolar patient are normally much lower than those of a average person, an "almost empty cash register" so to speak, the stress levels to "make one sick" (or not "make change") is at a much lower level than a person with normal kidney function.** This refers to our cash register analogy from chapter 5.

---

[157] http://www.duke.edu/~djs3/bio/

Upon stimulation by ACTH, the adrenal cortex secretes cortisol, a protein bound steroid. A deficiency in protein will result in higher levels of free cortisol. Cortisol is metabolized by 11-hydroxysteroid dehydrogenase to cortisone. Cortisol is synthesized from cholesterol. Increased cortisol can produce behavioral changes, increased stomach acid production, increased platelet production, increased red cell production. Cortisol has an affects vitamin D by increasing calcium absorption. Cortisol increases blood sugar levels usually in response to "fight or flight" scenarios. Stress can influence the secretion and duration of action of cortisol. Cortisol promotes catabolization of connective tissue and muscle. Cortisol requires 21-beta *hydroxylase* for synthesis. If cortisol is not synthesized, then biofeedback produces increased levels of ACTH to compensate. This results in adrenal hyperplasia and virilization.[158] My son showed significant signs of virilization.

- Cortisol defends the body against hypoglycaemia evoked by insulin.
- Cortisol stimulates hepatic glucose production (gluconeogenesis).
- Cortisol augments the glucagon stimulation of glycogenolysis.
- Cortisol inhibits the glucose uptake in target cells (GLUT 4 in muscle cells, heart cells and adipocytes).
- Cortisol is diabetogenic.

Cortisol antagonises the action of 1,25-dihydroxy-cholecalciferol and thus the absorption of Ca^{2+} from the gut—cortisol excess leads to osteoporosis.[159] **This explains the cause of psychosis.** Low normal mineral levels would be severely diminished by excessive cortisol production over a length of time. The result is vitamin pathway failures especially in the water-soluble vitamins thiamine, pyridoxine, and ascorbic acid. Notably, plasma cortisol levels increased significantly during metabolic acidosis but not during respiratory acidosis.[160]

Glucocorticoids induce phosphaturia, and decreased tubular reabsorption of phosphate has been reported 254 208. These effects can be attributed in large part to secondary hyperparathyroidism; however, glucocorticoids have also direct effects on the kidney.[161]

---

[158] http://www.pharmacology2000.com/Adrenocorticosteroids/physiol1.htm

[159] http://www.mfi.ku.dk/ppaulev/chapter30/Chapter%2030.htm

[160] http://ajpregu.physiology.org/cgi/content/full/277/2/R482

[161] http://www.endotext.com/adrenal/adrenal7/adrenalframe7.htm

Cortisol, a glucocorticoid, is secreted normally twice a day. The times are usually 4a.m. and 2p.m. These are also periods of significant sleep. If you experience significant "afternoon swoon" your phosphate levels are probably low.

Stress poses a dire threat to this body's minerals that are dangerously close to the edge from the start. Stress induced phosphaturia leads to increasing mineral losses with resulting vitamin pathway failures. As I see it there are two types of stress (1) real stress and (2) imagined stress. Real stress is obvious. A mountain lion attacks you in the wilderness. You (a) stand and fight or (b) run like hell. The body stimulates adrenaline and cortisol production so that you can survive. Imagined stress is probably what a psychologist would call neurosis. This is stress that *you place upon yourself*. In this case, you are actually in control. **It is very important for a bipolar person to know that he controls this stress and not the reverse.** A great example of a person who controlled stress was the founder of Wal-Mart. A few years ago, I read Sam Walton's response to a reporter who had asked Sam how he felt after Walmart stock had fallen substantially. He had personally lost over a billion dollars. Sam Walton's reply was that he was still alive and he had plenty of food to eat. In other words, he understood that this loss did not pose a personal threat. It was a part of playing the game in business. I am sure he was concerned about the loss of money, but life is going to have ups and downs. So look on the bright side. The energy spent on worrying is not going to change the scores on your college exams. Understand that the energy spent on stress usually only makes things worse.

I believe stress is related to resistance. This is the fight part of the equation. For example, if you remain in a job when you know you are not suited for that position, then you are resisting change. Ultimately stress is the result. In order to become more stress free it is imperative to learn to calculate how much energy should be put up for resistance and when is it time to change. As a general rule, it may be time to see the doctor if you are experiencing stress and your urine has developed an orange tint due to chromium loss.

The question that now comes to mind is "What causes psychosis?" I believe the answer is stress. Stress can bring down this house of cards in which a person with bipolar disease lives.

The adrenal glands are located just above the kidneys. The adrenal glands produce some very important compounds. During stress the adrenal medulla secretes epinephrine, the fight or flight neurotransmitter, a catecholamine. The adrenal cortex secretes glucocorticoids.

Physiological expenses for increased glucocorticoids levels include: Higher glucose levels, probably from glycolysis and gluconeogenesis, and increased blood pressure, probably from vasoconstriction. Decreased digestion, decreased immunity, probably from zinc loss and other factors, decreased

brain metabolism, probably from shunting in fight or flight preparation and decreased growth.

Chronic stress is implicated in diabetes, hypertension, heart disease, amenorrhea, and immunosuppression. Laboratory rats exposed to acute stress injected with nor-epinephrine produced increased retention of avoidance response.

Both the amygdala and the hippocampus, brain areas, have high levels of glucocorticoid receptors. The two types of receptors are (1) high affinity mineral corticoid receptors (MR's) and (2) low affinity glucocorticoid receptors (GR's). The hippocampus is involved in a negative feedback loop where it can shut down the response of the hippocampus after detecting high levels of glucocorticoids. This is known as the "deer in the headlights" effect.

Epinephrine produced by the adrenal medulla is detected by the vagus nerve which modulates hunger, satiety, vomiting, desire to urinate, stress, etc. The vagus nerve afferents that detect blood levels of epinephrine synapse on the nucleus of the solitary tract (NTS) in the medulla. Neurons for NTS project both to the amygdala and locus coerulus where they activate the nor-epinephrine system.

The amygdala is the brain system that is involved in the expression of emotions.
(1) Fear expression and evaluation
(2) Monitor emotions and modulation of memories.

There are 4 major modulator systems:
(1) Acetylcholine=modulates attention (pantothenic acid)
(2) Dopamine= modulates reinforcement (thiamine and pyridoxine)
(3) Nor epinephrine = stress (pyridoxine)
(4) Serotonin= mood (pyridoxine)

(I differ on number 4, because I consider GABA to play a very critical role in mood. GABA production depends on pyridoxine).

Glucocorticoids down regulates brain metabolism. The brain is a high-energy consumer. The hippocampus is sensitive to being deprived of energy that it needs for daily maintenance. Hypoglycemia, cholinergic and serotogenic toxins all lead to increased neuronal death coincidental with high glucocorticoid levels. (Therefore, attention deficits and mood instability would be expected). Glucocorticoids secreted during stress causes decreases in glucose brain up by up to 15 to 25 %. High glucocorticoids levels produce high glutamate levels. (A related compound, glutamine, is required for GABA production requiring pyridoxine). Glucocorticoids blunt GABA release. (This may be the result of shunting the pyridoxine catecholamine pathway toward NE production for use in the fight or flight response. This may result in fewer smiles). Stress produces decreased phosphate levels, which causes cation loss.[162]

Among the many mechanisms by which glucocorticoids induce osteoporosis (OP), a hyperparathyroid state is believed to be of critical importance.[163]

Cortisol is a glucocorticoid produced by the adrenal gland. **Cortisol is protein bound.** Cortisol's principle actions are to increase gluconeogenesis, glycogenolysis, and protein metabolism. These effects will increase glucose and ammonia levels.[164] **Remember bipolar people tend to have low levels of protein. This produces a condition of higher free cortisol.**

---

[162] http://socrates.berkeley.edu/~psy114/week14_lecture.html

[163] http://www.rheuma21st.com/archives/report_gio_int_cong_shoefeld_cutolo.html

[164] Harrison's Principles of Internal Medicine, 10th Edition, page 638.

STRESS INDUCED PSYCHOSIS

Stress induces inhibition of "active" vitamin D synthesis (bipolar mineral levels are low)

PSYCHOSIS

Phosphate loss

Magnesium deficiency fails causing excessive Chloride ion influx in nerve, "nerve excitation"

Loss of buffering capacity induces acidosis

Manganese deficiency = decreased GABA (well-being) and decreased vitamin K function (bleeding)

Chloride reabsorption

Overactive Sodium and Hydrogen exchange with Potassium, Minerals bind to excessive negative hydroxide ion and excreted

Glucose 6-deficiency causes "refeeding

Copper deficiency = tremor, insomnia, & anemia

Bicarbonate loss

tyrosine hydroxylase deficiency=dopamine deficiency

Vitamin failure

7-alpha hydroxylase deficiency down-regulates bile secretion causing malabsorption of bile cations, e.g. manganese and copper

Tryptophan hydroxylase failure=deficiencies of: melatonin (insomnia), serotonin (mood & awakening), dopamine ("overwhelmed" thoughts)

hypochlorhydria, decrease GI acidity, decreased iron absorption

These effects result in the following:

CHAPTER 30

Alcohol and Drug Abuse

"Fire and Rain"-Sweetbaby James

The refeeding syndrome from hypophosphatemia is a very strong pro-addictive force. I have experienced this in the form of sweet craving, rather than alcohol, and I have watched my son experience sweet craving, too. I believe that hypophosphatemia may play a very significant role in binge eating or drinking. This is especially true if the person, with relative frequency, eats a gallon of ice cream at a sitting or drinks a bottle of liquor. The refeeding syndrome is initiated by what I theorize are high ratios of cAMP to ATP.

Alcohol is pure carbohydrate (sugar). A bipolar person in a hypercatabolic or over-heated state tends to want to maintain that state. The alcoholic, for a reason that I have not determined, prefers alcohol as the carbohydrate of choice. A smoky, poorly ventilated bar would be the perfect place to maintain this state of glycolysis. Respiratory alkalosis and the enzyme phosphofructokinase are associated with glycolysis.

Magnesium and manganese convert alpha ketoglutamate to GABA, the "happy" neurotransmitter. Magnesium is protein bound. Bipolar people tend to have low protein levels. This low level of protein would result in more available magnesium for GABA production. This condition, along with magnesium, may explain why alcoholics do not get drunk. They probably started out feeling drunk when they originally started drinking. However, as the years went on they became protein deficient and mineral deficient, probably from dietary deficiency and physcial addiction to alcohol. Now, without enough magnesium to activate pyridoxine, they cannot convert alpha ketoglutamate to GABA, therefore, they no longer get drunk from alcohol.

Alcoholics tend to drink more during bouts of anger or depression. This could be caused from a stimulated stress-cortisol system producing phosphate depletion. *Glucocorticoids induce phosphaturia, and decreased tubular reabsorption of phosphate has been reported 254 208. These effects can be attributed in large part to secondary hyperparathyroidism; however, glucocorticoids have also direct effects on the kidney.*[165]

Because of the decreased level of bicarbonate and resulting decrease in buffering capacity bipolar people would tend to become angrier more easily than a normal person. Because of the acidosis induced magnesium loss the production of GABA would be decreased resulting in depression or anxiety. The result may be "I need a drink."

One's choice of spirits may tell a lot about how you have learned to cope. For example, scotch whiskey contains a high level of manganese. Manganese as we have seen is good for mood. The combination of the two probably produces a generally happy alcoholic. A drink that contains seltzer water, which contains bicarbonate may make this person may feel cool and calm. Similarly, beer is derived from grain, which would contain magnesium and manganese and may be carbonated as well. A drink called screwdriver has vodka and orange juice. The o.j. would provide potassium. The same could be said for the bloody mary, which contains tomato juice, which is also high in potassium. A person drinking vodka on the rocks would be expected to have a very serious drink problem.

Alcohol decreases ADH release causing increased urinary volume, which causes increased phosphate loss. This produces energy loss and a decreased ability to buffer, which makes you more susceptible to stress. Alcohol decreases levels of sodium while increasing levels of potassium. **Hyperventilation produces glucose breakdown resulting in hypophosphatemia.**

Prolonged rapid, shallow breathing results in excessive loss of carbon dioxide and decreased blood acidity (i.e., alkalosis), which in turn activates an enzyme that enhances glucose breakdown. In glucose breakdown, phosphate becomes incorporated into various metabolic compounds, ultimately lowering blood levels of phosphate. As the rate of glucose breakdown increases, profound hypophosphatemia potentially can result.[166] Alcohol intake should be limited because ethanol will reduce osteoblastic activity, lower parathyroid hormone (PTH) levels, and contribute to osteoporosis. It also indirectly accelerates osteoclastic activity, increases urinary calcium excretion, and contributes to bone loss.[167]

---

[165] http://www.endotext.com/adrenal/adrenal7/adrenalframe7.htm
[166] http://www.niaaa.nih.gov/publications/arh21-1/84.pdf
[167] http://author.emedicine.com/MED/topic1069.htm

Acute alcohol ingestion causes **hypoparathyroidism** with hypercalciuria and hypocalcemia. PTH levels can drop by 70% after acute alcohol intoxication. Prolonged but moderate alcohol intake eventually will raise PTH levels. People with chronic alcoholism develop low serum vitamin D levels, which cause impaired intestinal calcium absorption and hypocalciuria. A direct inhibitory effect on osteoblast activity by alcohol ingestion also appears to exist. This effect is enhanced in smokers. Urinary calcium excretion during periods of alcohol consumption can increase by over 200% over controls. Osteopenia also has been linked to alcohol consumption.[168] This decrease in PTH probably makes the bipolar person feel more "normal" initially.

Many bipolar people, to "quite their nerves," use alcohol, but it actually disturbs sleep by its effect on REM. Alcohol is also a carbohydrate (a sugar).

Cocaine prolongs the effect of dopamine in the synapses. [169] This may partly explain drug abuse in bipolar people. Dopamine synthesis depends on copper. We have shown that copper levels in bipolar patients could be low and, therefore, dopamine levels would be low as well. In the short term, cocaine may actually make this type of person feel better. This may initially entice a dopamine deficient person into continued use. The results can be disastrous.

It is important to note that **nicotine is a potent stimulant of tyrosine hydroxylase**.[170] **Morphine and cocaine are also potent stimulants of tyrosine hydroxylase**.[171] Since these drugs are commonly abused by people with mental illness this would lead to an assumption that other hydroxylase pathways should be monitored. Could it be that these drugs actually make this person feel more normal? After continued use of a potent drug one would expect the enzyme and/or catalyst to be excessively used and depleted resulting in drug failure. The physical condition should be worse than before drug use. An abundance of substrate at this enzyme bottleneck may result in toxic effects. I have little experience with people who abuse drugs and this theory has just evolved from research.

I have no scientific proof, just personal observation, that some video games produce high stress levels. Video games provide immediate feedback and performance requires extremely high attention. This chronically heightened attention probably leads to deficiency of acetylcholine produced by pantothenic acid.

---

[168] http://author.emedicine.com/MED/topic1069.htm

[169] http://unc.edu/~eckerman/P10drugs.html

[170] http://ajpcell.physiology.org/cgi/content/full/276/1/C54

[171] http://www.jneurosci.org/cgi/content/full/18/23/9989

A person playing these games continuously may experience attention deficits and dilated pupils. I expect that continued on the edge stress production will lead to high cortisol levels. This continual high level of cortisol will affect the body and mind. The high cortisol levels may blunt GABA production by stressing the pyridoxine-catecholamine pathway resulting in agitation and fewer smiles. In addition, sitting in a closed, poorly ventilated room with a device that emits heat and some gases for hours on hours will probably aid the development of glycolysis. Once the glycolysis starts it certainly seems that the attention deficits will follow.

I am not an advocate of abolition of video games. However, I do believe that the games should have built-in daily time limits. For example, after 2 hours the game shuts down until the next day. Parents have busy schedules and teenagers are frequently left to their own devices. A time limit would resolve some of these issues. This would allow the video game producers to still supply their product while protecting the public from themselves.

CHAPTER 31

Suicide

The second leading cause of death...

Why do people commit suicide? I do not know. I suspect it has to due with a lack of hope if it is a suicide with depression involvement or self-perception as a failure. I believe part of the dynamics of suicide involve energy. I have heard about people who are about to commit suicide start feeling better prior to the act. Why? From a very simplistic view, the obsessing about suicide must generate a great deal of stress. As we have seen, the negative effect on energy levels because of excessive phosphate excretion would mire a person in the muck of depression. A depressed person who makes a conscious decision to commit suicide has resolution. Resolution is a great stress reliever. As this depressed person's energy levels rise while still in a depressed state, then the act may take place. Unlike the person with mania who gets an extremely rapid rise in energy levels through direct action by phosphate reabsorption, these people may only see a mild to moderate rise in energy levels. This may be just enough energy to commit suicide. A psychotic suicide is very different from a depression suicide. This is because the psychotic is confused and they are reacting out of fear.

I found a very good source that describes some of the symptoms of potential suicide. This source is the National Association of Mental Health.

In 1996, more teenagers and young adults died of suicide than from cancer, heart disease, AIDS, birth defects, stroke, pneumonia and influenza, and chronic lung disease **combined.**

In 1996, suicide was the <u>second-leading cause of death among college students, the third-leading cause of death among those aged 15 to 24 years, and the fourth-leading cause of death among those aged 10 to 14 years.</u>

Suicide "Signs"

There are many behavioral indicators that can help parents or friends recognize the threat of suicide in a loved one. Since mental and substance-related disorders so frequently accompany suicidal behavior, many of the cues to be looked for are symptoms associated with such disorders as depression, bipolar disorder (manic depression), anxiety disorders, alcohol and drug use, disruptive behavior disorders, borderline personality disorder, and schizophrenia.

Some common symptoms of these disorders include:
- Extreme personality changes
- Loss of interest in activities that used to be enjoyable
- Significant loss or gain in appetite
- Difficulty falling asleep or wanting to sleep all day
- Fatigue or loss of energy
- Feelings of worthlessness or guilt
- Withdrawal from family and friends
- Neglect of personal appearance or hygiene
- Sadness, irritability, or indifference
- Having trouble concentrating
- Extreme anxiety or panic
- Drug or alcohol use or abuse
- Aggressive, destructive, or defiant behavior
- Poor school performance
- Hallucinations or unusual beliefs

Tragically, many of these signs go unrecognized. Suffering from one of these symptoms does not necessarily mean that one is suicidal, it's always best to communicate openly with a loved one who has one or more of these behaviors, especially if they are unusual for that person.

There are also some more obvious signs of the potential for committing suicide. Putting one's affairs in order, such as giving or throwing away favorite belongings, is a strong clue. And it can't be stressed more strongly that any talk of death or suicide should be taken seriously and paid close attention to. It is a sad fact that while many of those who commit suicide talked about it beforehand, only 33 percent to 50 percent were identified by their doctors as having a mental illness at the time of their death and only 15 percent of suicide victims were in treatment at the time of their death. Any history of previous suicide attempts is also reason for concern and watchfulness. Approximately one-third of teens that die by suicide have made a previous suicide attempt. It should be noted as well that while more females attempt suicide, more males are success-ful in completing suicide.

Causes

While the reasons that teens commit suicide vary widely, there are some common situations and circumstances that seem to lead to such extreme measures. These include major disappointment, rejection, failure, or loss such as breaking up with a girlfriend or boyfriend, failing a big exam, or witnessing family turmoil. Since the overwhelming majority of those who commit suicide have a mental or substance-related disorder, they often have difficulty coping with such crippling stressors. They are unable to see that their life can turn around, unable to recognize that suicide is a permanent solution to a tempo-rary problem. Usually, the common reasons for suicide listed above are actu-ally not the "causes" of the suicide, but rather triggers for suicide in a person suffering from a mental illness or substance-related disorder.

More recently, scientists have focused on the biology of suicide. Suicide is thought by some to have a genetic component, to run in families. And research has shown strong evidence that mental and substance-related disorders, which commonly affect those who end up committing suicide, do run in families. While the suicide of a relative is obviously not a direct "cause" of suicide, it does, perhaps, put certain individuals at more risk than others. Certainly, the suicide of one's parent or other close family member could lead to thoughts of such behavior in a teen with a mental or substance-related disorder.

Research has also explored the specific brain chemistry of those who take their own lives. Recent studies indicate that those who have attempted suicide may also have low levels of the brain chemical serotonin. Serotonin helps control impulsiv-ity, and low levels of the brain chemical are thought to cause more impulsive behavior. Suicides are often committed out of impulse. Antidepressant drugs affecting serotonin are used to treat depression, impulsivity, and suicidal thoughts. However, much more research is needed to confirm these hypotheses and, hopefully, eventually lead to more definite indicators of and treatment for those prone to suicide.

How to Help

Since people who are contemplating suicide feel so alone and helpless, the most important thing to do if you think a friend or loved one is suicidal is to com-municate with him or her openly and frequently. Make it clear that you care; stress your willingness to listen. Also, be sure to take all talk of suicide seriously.

Don't assume that people who talk about killing themselves won't really do it. An estimated 80 percent of all those who commit suicide give some warning of their intentions or mention their feelings to a friend or family member. Don't ignore what may seem like casual threats or remarks. Statements like "You'll be sorry when I'm dead" and "I can't see any way out," no matter how off-the-cuff or jokingly said, may indicate serious suicidal feelings.

One of the most common misconceptions about talking with someone who might be contemplating suicide is that bringing up the subject may make things worse. This is **not** true. There is no danger of "giving someone the idea." Rather, the opposite is correct. Bringing up the question of suicide and discussing it without showing shock or disapproval is one of the most helpful things you can do. This openness shows that you are taking the individual seriously and responding to the severity of his or her distress.

If you do find that your friend or loved one is contemplating suicide, it is essential to help him or her find immediate professional care. (**Calling the NAMI HelpLine at 1-800-950-NAMI [6264]** for more information or to help you locate your local NAMI for area assistance is one possible resource). Don't make the common misjudgment that those contemplating suicide are unwilling to seek help. Studies of suicide victims show that more than half had sought medical help within six months before their deaths. And don't leave the suicidal person to find help alone—they usually aren't capable. Also, **never** assume that someone who is determined to end his or her life can't be stopped. Even the most severely depressed person has mixed feelings about death, wavering until the very last moment between wanting to live and wanting to die. Most suicidal people do not want death; they want the pain to stop. The impulse to end it all, though, no matter how overpowering, does not last forever.

If the threat is immediate, if your friend or loved one tells you he or she is going to commit suicide, you must act immediately. Don't leave the person alone, and don't try to argue. Instead, ask questions like, "Have you thought about how you'd do it?" "Do you have the means?" and "Have you decided when you'll do it?" If the person has a defined plan, the means are easily available, the method is a lethal one, and the time is set, the risk of suicide is obviously severe. In such an instance, you **must** take the individual to the nearest psychiatric facility or hospital emergency room. If you are together on the phone, you may even need to call 911 or the police. Remember, under such circumstances no actions on your part should be considered too extreme—you are trying to save a life. Overwhelming majorities of young people who hear a suicide threat from a friend or loved one don't report the threat to an adult. Take all threats seriously—you are not betraying someone's trust by trying to keep them alive. **Other Serious Considerations**

Don't automatically assume that someone who was considering suicide and is now in treatment or tells you that he or she is feeling better is, in fact, doing better. Some who commit suicide actually do so just as they seem to be improving. One reason for this may be that they did not have enough energy to kill themselves when they were extremely depressed, but now has just enough energy to go through with their plan. Another reason for suicide during a seeming improvement is that resigning oneself to death can release anxiety. While it's not good to monitor every action of someone who is recovering from suicidal thoughts, it is important to make certain that the lines of communication between you and the individual remain open.

While it may seem a bit obvious, it should also be mentioned that it is extremely advisable to bar teens that are suicidal from access to firearms. Nearly 60 percent of all completed suicides are committed with a firearm. And while having a firearm does not in itself promote suicidal behavior, knowing that one is accessible may help a troubled teen formulate his or her suicidal plans.[172]

Besides the extreme social environment during the teen years, I have noted the tremendous change in skeletal structure especially in boys. This over-night change from a boy to a man creates a brand new metabolic dynamic. Nutritional demands change almost overnight. This new body requires a much larger quantities of minerals to run vitamin pathways. A deficient skeleton places this person at nutritional risk. I do not think these nutritional needs are being supplied to our American teenagers. Teachers should be educated about at-risk suicidal behaviors in order to establish parental contact to convey concern.

Social stresses can be extreme in a teen. It is of utmost importance that this person has adequate positive "stress relieving" support from his family and peers. Stress-cortisol related energy losses would continue in a teen that sits on a crumbling nutritional precipice. A tired, sleepy, and short-tempered teen will almost certainly find him friendless and devoid of hope. This is a recipe for suicide.

Although the dynamic physical changes have subsided by the college years, the pressure of academic and social life, coupled with alcohol and drugs, certainly create an environment conducive to suicide. Educating incoming freshman to the

---

[172] http://namiwi.nami.org/helpline/teensuicide.html

signs and behaviors of at-risk students is a good idea. On-campus support groups may be helpful.

I purchased the book, <u>The Bipolar Child</u>, by authors Papolos & Papolos. The authors mention studies of the Amish. The Amish are studied widely because they are essentially a closed society. Therefore, there is little variation in the genes. They say, "Few Amish children who go on to develop bipolar disorder are reported to have the same early co morbid conditions. For example separation anxiety, symptoms of attention-deficit disorder with hyperactivity, and oppositional defiant behaviors are uncommon. While anger dyscontrol and bossiness are frequently present in the Amish bipolar children, the degree and intensity of these symptoms seem markedly temperered.

The regularity and simplicity of the Amish lifestyle, characterized by consistent social values, a philosophy of nonviolence, strong family and community kinship structures, and a proscribed daily, weekly, and monthly schedule centering around the church provide focus and structure to the social world. The absence of electricity wed the Amish to the natural daily and seasonal light/dark cycles, and in-comparison to the ordinary American child-introduces a complete buffer to over stimulation."[173]

This passage mentions everything but diet. The Amish probably eat organically grown foods. Therefore, they would avoid much of the mercury toxicity that society is exposed. The foods they eat are probably nutrient rich, rather than the depleted variety that society eats. The probably have never had a Twinkie. The milk they drink is probably straight from the cow; no vitamin D added. Their environment is as stress-free as any in the world. An Amish lifestyle is probably a very healthy one for the bipolar population.

---

[173] The Bipolar Child, Demitri Papolos and Janice Papolos, page 165.

CHAPTER 32

Other Factors

Synthetic bipolar disease

Topiramate

Why does this drug produce a bipolar-like syndrome? It appears that the side effects of this drug go a long way in proving my theory. Recently, I received a letter from the manufacturer of the anticonvulsant topiramate warning of the potential for topiramate to produce metabolic acidosis. Specifically, the manufacturer states that **topiramate produces hyperchloremic, non-anion gap metabolic acidosis due to decreases in bicarbonate production due to carbonic anhydrase inhibition. Note that anticonvulsants, in general, antagonize the effect of vitamin D.** It is therefore possible that this antagonism may be caused by interference with 1 alpha hydroxylase, the enzyme necessary to activate 1, 25 DHCC. This interference is linked to carbonic anhydrase inhibition. Fatigue, anorexia, and growth reduction are common side effects of this drug. **Psychological disorders associated with this disease include excessive sleep, nervousness, memory loss, anorexia, confusion, depression, attention deficits, mood swings, and speech disorder (word finding difficulties).**

Also, a condition of acute myopia (nearsightedness) associated with secondary angle closure glaucoma has been reported.[174]

Note the similarities between the psychological disorders and bipolar disease. Also, note the nearsightedness, which I believe, is a common finding among people with bipolar disease.

---

[174] http://www.fda.gov/medwatch.SAFETY/2003/topamax

MERCURY

The heavy metal mercury is frequently in the news being linked to tuna and other fish. What effects does mercury have on the body? **Mercury can cause an extremely high production of glutamate.** As we have seen, the expectation would be attention deficits. This excess glutamate is converted to glutamine and ammonia ion. Ammonia ion is by itself a neurotoxin. The body also responds to the high glutamate levels by producing secretin, a hormone for stomach acid production, which increases chances for gastrointestinal diseases. Mercury also acts on the kidney producing potassium and magnesium losses. Amalgam fillings used by dentists in earlier times contained mercury. A older bipolar patient is likely to have many of these because of cavities produced by sweet craving producing acids, bone dissolution, and dry mouth. **The side effects of mercury poisoning are insomnia, shyness, emotional instability, memory loss, depression, anorexia, excessive perspiration, blushing, tremors, gingivitis, salivation, and hearing loss.** [175] Some diuretics are mercury based. Seeing a professional about toxicity associated with mercury may be recommended in some extreme cases. Although mercury is very difficult to eliminate from the body some physicians are chelating it with success.

AMINO ACIDS

These amino acids may be involved in some way but they have not been investigated. Tyrosine is involved in renal tubular dysfunction. Glycine is associated with renal failure. Cysteine is involved in Fanconi syndrome, renal tubular disorder, and proximal renal tubular swan neck. Lysine and arginine are associated with metabolic acidosis. [176] I provided this for information purposes I have not studied these amino acids, but I found their relation to the topic warranted inclusion.

---

[175] http://cdc.gov epidemiologic notes and reports elemental mercury poisoning
[176] Harrison's Principles of Internal Medicine, 10th Edition, page 511.

Chapter 33

Vitamin Reference

"Vita-Vega Vitamin, Lucy"

THIAMINE diphosphate, VITAMIN B-1, Magnesium and Copper

Thiamine diphosphate is important in carbohydrate, sugars and starches, metabolism. Thiamine requires either the element magnesium or copper as catalysts or metallic co-factors. The failure to reabsorb phosphate ion in the kidney leads to excessive phosphate lost in urination. This ultimately leads to low phosphate levels in the body. This factor would slow down the rate of thiamine related metabolic reactions. However, if this deficiency is coupled with a mineral deficiency also, then the thiamine pathway loses on both ends. Phosphate ion is extremely important for energy production. This low phosphate level causes the body to crave carbohydrates. Thiamine is involved in carbohydrate metabolism.[177]

People with bipolar disease tend to be carbohydrate "hogs". That is, they crave ravenously sugars, starches, or, and yes, alcohol. A normal person would be satisfied once the blood sugar and phosphate levels were restored. However, since phosphate ion is depleted this condition continues on and on, therefore, re-feeding. *Thiamine requirement must be proportional to calories ingestion.*[178] Therefore, a person craving carbohydrates would be thiamine stressed. As you can see, the maintenance of thiamine level would be difficult in this re-feeding

---

[177] The Merck Manual, 15th Edition, 1987, page 932.
[178] Harrison's Principles of Internal Medicine, 10th Edition.

syndrome. This may explain the genetic link to Glucose 6-Phosphate deficiency in bipolar disease.

Thiamine specifically acts to decarboxylate alpha keto acids (pyuvate and alpha ketoglutarate).[179] This is especially important in regards to "mood" in that alpha ketoglutamate is converted to gamma amino butyric acid or GABA, which provides a "feeling of well being." The element magnesium is necessary to catalyze this chemical reaction. Thiamine is also involved in metabolism of the amino acids leucine, isoleucine, and valine. Note that the disorder of leucine catabolism produces "sweaty feet" odor and metabolic ketoacidosis.[180]

Failure of the thiamine pathway results in fatigue, irritation, and poor memory. Large amounts of thiamine are present in skeletal muscles, heart, liver, kidneys, and brain. Thiamine is absorbed actively and passively from the gut. [181]

Sleep disturbances occur because a deficiency of thiamine or co-factor copper prevents the conversion of tryptophan to melatonin. Melatonin is necessary for sleep production. Constipation may also occur possibly due to depleted energy levels from extremely low phoshate levels. Numbness or tingling in the hands or feet is also a symptom of thiamine defiency. Anorexia is also mentioned.[182]

The medical name for thiamine deficiency is Beri-beri. There are two types of Beriberi, cerebral and cardiovascular, head and heart, also known as dry beriberi and wet beriberi respectively. "Three types of nervous system involvement occur: peripheral neuropathy, Wernicke's encephalopathy, (cerebral beriberi), and the Korsakoff syndrome." Cerebral beriberi produces mental confusion, aphonia (decreased vocal sounds), CONFABULATION (a mixture of symptoms including MANIA AND DEPRESSION), decreased cerebral blood flow, increased vascular resistance (blood pressure), and nystagmus (an eye condition). Other symptoms are retrograde amnesia, impaired ability to learn, non-inflammatory degeneration of myelin sheath. Cardiovascular or wet beriberi "comprises three major physiologic derangements: (1) peripheral vasodilatation leading to a high-output state, (2) biventricular myocardial failure, and (3) retention of sodium and water leading to edema." Note the symptom "stocking glove cyanosis"[183].

---

[179] The Merck Manual, 15th Edition, 1987, page 932.

[180] Harrison's Principles of Internal Medicine, 10th Edition.

[181] The Merck Manual, 15th Edition, 1987, page 932.

[182] The Merck Manual, 15th Edition, 1987, page 932.

[183] Harrison's Principles of Internal Medicine, 10th Edition.

"Severe physical exertion, high carbohydrate intake, and a moderate degree of chronic deficiency favor wet beriberi."[184] Be aware that this could occur in athletes would ingest large amounts of soft drinks. "Subjective symptoms include generalized malaise, headache, nausea, and aching of muscles." Cardiovascular or wet beriberi symptoms include tachycardia (fast heart rate), sweating, warm skin, cold and cyanotic extremities (blue toes or fingers), and slow reflexes.[185] Magnesium is a co-factor for transketolase. "Development of these symptoms is paralleled by a fall in red blood cell transketolase activity."[186]

Thiamine diphosphate, magnesium and copper are very important pieces to this bipolar puzzle. Copper and thiamine help induce sleep. Insomnia is a critical symptom of bipolar illness. Sleep deprivation can lead to psychosis. Magnesium and thiamine are necessary for a good mood.

Hallmark signs of thiamine deficiency include fatigue, irritation, poor memory, mania and depression (confabulation), stocking glove cyanosis, sweating, warm skin, and carbohydrate cravings.[187] Note that these coincide with those of bipolar disease. It is very important that a person with bipolar disease recognize these symptoms in order to take steps to correct this deficiency. Note that alcohol decreases thiamine absorption. Thiamine is secreted by renal tubules.

RIBOFLAVIN, Iron or Nickel or Molydenum

Riboflavin is involved in oxidative-reduction reactions. Riboflavin requires iron or nickel as a co-factor. Deficiency includes oral, ocular, cutaneous (skin), and genital lesions. Primary deficiency may occur from inadequate consumption of milk and other animal protein. Symptoms of riboflavin deficiency include pallor (pale), *lesions in the angles of the mouth*, and magenta tongue. Sunlight produces riboflavin destruction. Therefore it may be wise to supplement riboflavin before sunbathing. Riboflavin is necessary for niacin production along with vitamin B1 and vitamin B6.[188]

---

184 Harrison's Principles of Internal Medicine, 10th Edition
185 Harrison's Principles of Internal Medicine, 10th Edition
186 Harrison's Principles of Internal Medicine, 10th Edition
187 The Merck Manual, 15th Edition, 1987, page 932.
188 The Merck Manual, 15th Edtion, 1987, page 933.

PYRIDOXINE Phosphate, VITAMIN B6, CHROMIUM AND MAGNESIUM

Pyridoxine is involved in decarboxylation and transamination of amino acis, deamination of hydroxyamines acids and cysteine. Vitamin B6 is metabolized to niacin. Vitamin B6 is involved in the metabolism of fatty acids. Vitamin B6 is important in the blood, CNS, and skin. A SECONDARY DEFICIENCY OF VITAMIN B6 INCREASES METABOLIC ACTIVITY.

Vitamin B6 deficiency can produce "lymphopenia" and convulsions. Vitamin B6 is water-soluble. Water-soluble vitamins need to be replenished frequently during the day.[189]

Vitamin B6 functions as a co-enzyme for glycogen phosphorylase, an enzyme that catalyzes the release of glucose stores in muscle as glycogen (glycolysis!). Vitamin B6 is used to generate glucose from amino acids "gluconeogenesis".[190] (The failure to generate glucose through glucoenogenesis may be the reason for carbohydrate cravings in bipolar people).

Vitamin B6 synthesizes tryptophan to serotonin and is metabolized to niacin in the process. Vitamin B6 is involved in the synthesis of dopamine, NE, and GABA. Vitamin B6 is involved in hemoglobin production. Vitamin B6 may decrease the effect of steroid hormones by binding steroid receptor sites. Vitamin B6 deficiency produces irritability, depression, confusion, mouth ulcers, increased dietary protein causes increased vitamin B6 requirement. Homocysteine, a compound linked to atherosclerosis and stress, conversion is regulated by folic acid, B12, and B6. High doses of vitamin B6 decreases the incidence of kidney stones.[191]

The catecholamines norepinephrine, epinephrine, and dopamine are produced in the adrenal glands. Vitamin B6 helps synthesize the inhibitory neurotransmitter dopamine. Dopamine modulates reinforcement and filters stimuli. Vitamin B6 helps synthesize norepinephrine, NE, which modulates stress. Vitamin B6 helps synthesize the inhibitory neurotransmitter GABA that is generally recognized as the compound that produces the feeling of well-being.

Dopaminergic receptors utilize the adenyl-cyclase cyclic AMP system as a second messenger.[192] Note that because of phosphate depletion the level of cyclic AMP may be higher in bipolar people.

---

[189] The Merck Manual, 15th Edtion, 1987, page 933.

[190] http://lpi.oregonstate.edu/infocenter/pyridoxine/html.

[191] http://lpi.oregonstate.edu/infocenter/pyridoxine/html

[192] Harrison's Principles of Internal Medicine, 10th Edition, page 412.

Harrison's also mentions, *"By direct action in the renal tubule, cate-cholamines stimulate <u>sodium reabsorption</u>, thereby, defending extracellular fluid volume. Catecholamines also promote cellular uptake of potassium, thereby defending against the development of hyperkalemia."*[193]

Vitamin B6 may improve the effectiveness of cation tricyclic antidepressants.[194] MAOI's, another form of antidepressant, may reduce blood levels of vitamin B6 possibly from stimulating vitamin B6 actions and metabolism. There is evidence vitamin B6 may help with ADHD (attention deficit hyperactive disorder). Vitamin B6 may possibly help with diabetes. Pyridine therapy appears to be an effective and appropriate strategy to ameliorate plasma homocysteine, triglyceridemia, and total choldesterol levels in patients with chronic renal failure who are reliably known to be at risk for atherosclerosis.[195]

The mechanism of action of vitamin B6 involves transaminases, synthetases, and **hydroxylases**.[196] NOTE THAT WE ARE SPECIFICALLY CONCERNED ABOUT 1 ALPHA HYDROXYLASE. Vitamin B6 is involved in metabolism of tryptophan, glycine, serine, glutamate, and sulfur containing amino acids. Vitamin B6 is involved in the synthesis of the heme precursor gamma amino levulinic acid.[197]

Vitamin B6 is involved in enzymes known as dehydrogenases. Vitamin B6 appears to involve in the splitting of water into hydrogen and hydroxide ions. In the case of vitamin pathway failure these ions would not be formed and inadequate bicarbonate formation would occur. The combination of inadequate phosphate reabsorption and inadequate bicarbonate formation results in a significant decrease in the body's ability to buffer acids.

FOLIC ACID, Zinc

Folic acid is responsible for one-carbon transfers in purine and pyridine (protein) metabolism. Anemia may result from deficiency. Folic acid is involved in DNA synthesis and the synthesis of S-adenosylmethionine or SAM. SAM has been purported to play a key role in mood. Folic acid is found

---

[193] Harrison's Principles of Internal Medicine, 10th Edition, page413.

[194] http://www.umm.edu/pyridoxine/html.

[195] http://www.umm.edu/pyridoxine/html.

[196] Harrison's Principles of Internal Medicine, 10th Edition, page 465.

[197] Harrison's Principles of Internal Medicine, 10th Edition, page 465.

in large amounts in the brain and heart. Folic acid is involved in conversion of homocysteine into methionine.

Homocysteine is a risk factor in heart disease and Alzheimer disease. Therefore, a deficiency in folic acid may result in higher levels of homocysteine, which may have deleterious effects on the heart and the brain, especially the hippocampus. Stress tends to increase levels of homocysteine.

Folic acid requirement is increased by alcohol. Serine, the amino acid, interacts with zinc and folate to produce glycine. Glycine acts as an inhibitory second messenger in the brain.[198]

CYANOCOBALAMIN, VITAMIN B-12, Cobalt

Cyanocobalamin or vitamin B-12 requires the mineral cobalt to be effective. Vitamin B-12 facilitates the reduction of ribose to help with DNA synthesis. Vitamin B-12 works with vitamin B-6, folic acid and zinc to decrease homocysteine (stress). Vitamin B-12 is important for DNA and RNA, energy production form fats and proteins (glycolysis and gluconeogenesis), hemoglobin synthesis (blood), and for the treatment of pernicious anemia. Vitamin B-12 is secreted by the *parietal cells* of the gastric mucosa (stomach).

Neurologic symptoms include: (1) peripheral neuropathy, (2) difficulty walking, (3) memory loss, (4) disorientation, (5) dementia with or without mood change, and (6) poor finger coordination. Vitamin B-12 deficiency may cause myelin sheath damage. Only bacteria can synthesize vitamin B-12.[199]

Food sources include *clams, crab, salmon, beef chicken, turkey, eggs, and milk Vitamin B-12 is available in a prescription inject able form, a nasal gel, a sublingual solution, and a tablet (tablets tend not to be absorbed).

BIOTIN, Magnesium and Manganese

Biotin regulates metabolism of both fat and carbohydrate. A deficiency results in retarded physical and mental development. Deficiency produces defective T cell and B cell immunity.[200] Biotin requires magnesium and manganese as

---

[198] The Merck Manual, 15 Edition, 1987, page 934.
[199] The Merck Manual, 15 Edition, 1987, page 937.
[200] The Merck Manual, 15th Edition, 1987, page 939.

co-factors. Biotin carboxylates fat and carbohydrate substrates producing Acetyl-CoA carboxylase for fatty acid synthesis, private carboxyalse for gluco-neogenesis, methylcrotonyl-CoA carboxylase for leucine metabolism, propri-onyl-CoA carboxylase for amino acid, cholesterol and fatty acid metabolism.[201]

Symptoms of deficiency include hair loss, scaly red rash around eyes, nose mouth, and genitalia. (Supplementation of biotin and pyridoxine, which blocks steroid receptor sites may help, reduce hair loss). CNS symptoms of deficiency include depression, lethargy, hallucination and peripheral numbness.

Biotin stimulates glucokinase in the liver promoting glycogen synthesis. Therefore, biotin deficiency may result in glycolysis or the breakdown of stored fat for energy consumption.[202] Glycolysis is a hallmark sign for phosphate defi-ciency. Food sources include baker's yeast, wheat bran, eggs, bread, and cheese.[203]

ASCORBIC ACID, VITAMIN C, IRON AND COPPER

Vitamin C is involved with the immune system. Vitamin C is needed for white cell function. Vitamin C is needed also for energy. It is needed for con-version of lysine to carnitine. Carnitine is necessary as muscle fuel. Vitamin C is needed for serotonin and melatonin production as well as dopamine and NE production. Vitamin C deficiency may result in sleep disturbances and possi-bly depression. Vitamin C is needed to produce cortisol and adrenalin. Vitamin C acts as an antioxidant and metal scavenger. Vitamin C is involved in tissue repair and vitamin C deficiency may result in bruises and bleeding gums. Vitamin C acts as to stimulate hydroxylase.[204]

PANTOTHENIC ACID, Magnesium and Manganese

The metallic co-enzyme for the vitamin Pantothenic acid appears to mag-nesium and manganese. Pantothenic acid is an essential component of co-enzyme A. Pantothenic acid provides the acyltransfer cofactor for many enzymatic reactions. Pantothenic acid is involved in the producton of acetyl-choline, melatonin and heme.

---

[201] http://lpi.oregonstate.edu/infocenter/biotin/html
[202] The Merck Manual, 15th Edition, 1987, page 939.
[203] http://lpi.oregonstate.edu/infocenter/biotin/html
[204] The Merck Manual, 15th Edition, 1987, page 940.

Acetylcholine is an important central excitatory neurotransmitter that monitors a person's attention, melatonin is involved with sleep, and heme is involved in blood formation. Pyridoxine is also involved in heme formation. *Acetylcholine stimulates ADH synthesis*, antidiuretic hormone, which prevents excessive urinary excretion, production, occurs in the SON (supra orbital nucleus of the eye).

Pantothenic acid is involved with manganese in cholesterol production and steroid synthesis. A deficiency results in "burning feet", decreased exercise tolerance, decreased glycogen, and decreased myelin sheath.

The derivative pantothenate has cholesterol-lowering effects. Food sources include: fish, tuna, chicken, egg, milk, bread, and yogurt. [205]

Z-BEC

The most important vitamins in this disease are thiamine or vitamin B-1, pyridoxine or vitamin B-6, and ascorbic acid or vitamin C. They are the big three. I get these vitamins by using a vitamin supplement that does not contain vitamin D. This product is called Z-Bec. This product contains zinc, vitamin E, vitamin B complex, and vitamin C all in high concentration. I receive no compensation from the makers of Z-Bec. I take this supplement twice a day, morning and afternoon. Zinc interferes with copper absorption so I do not take this vitamin after 5 p.m. I take copper and thiamine at bedtime for sleep induction.

---

[205] The Merck Manual, 15th Edition, 1987, page 939.

CHAPTER 34

Mineral Toxicities

Special Thanks to Linus Pauling Institute

Calcium

Toxicity

Abnormally elevated blood calcium (hypercalcemia) resulting from the over consumption of calcium has never been documented to occur from foods, only from calcium supplements. Mild hypercalcemia may be without symptoms, or may result in loss of appetite, nausea, vomiting, constipation, abdominal pain, dry mouth, thirst, and frequent urination. More severe hypercalcemia may result in confusion, delirium, coma, and if not treated, death. Hypercalcemia has been reported only with the consumption of large quantities of calcium supplements usually in combination with antacids, particularly in the days when peptic ulcers were treated with large quantities of milk, calcium carbonate (antacid) and sodium bicarbonate (absorbable alkali) (1). This condition was termed milk alkali syndrome, and has been reported at calcium supplement levels from 1.5 to 16.5 grams/day for 2 days to 30 years. Since the treatment for peptic ulcers has changed, the incidence of this syndrome has decreased considerably (3).

Although the risk of forming kidney stones is increased in individuals with abnormally elevated urinary calcium (hypercalciuria), this condition is not usually related to calcium intake, but rather to increased excretion of calcium by the kidneys. Overall, increased dietary calcium has been associated with a decreased risk of kidney stones. However, in a large prospective study, the risk of developing kidney stones in women taking supplemental calcium was 20% higher than in those who did not (21). This effect may be related to the fact that calcium supplements can be taken without food, eliminating their beneficial effect of decreasing intestinal oxalate absorption.

Based on the adverse effects above, as well as the potential for decreased absorption of other essential minerals (see below), the Food and Nutrition

Board of the Institute of Medicine set the tolerable upper level (UL) of intake for calcium in adults at 2,500 milligrams (mg) of calcium/day (3).

Chromium

Toxicity

Hexavalent chromium or chromium (VI) is a recognized carcinogen. Exposure to chromium (VI) in dust is associated with increased incidence of lung cancer and is known to cause inflammation of the skin (dermatitis). In contrast, there is little evidence that trivalent chromium or chromium (III) is toxic to humans. Because no adverse effects have been convincingly associated with excess intake of chromium (III) from food or supplements, the Food and Nutrition Board (FNB) of the Institute of Medicine did not set a tolerable upper level of intake (UL) for chromium. Because information is limited, the FNB acknowledged a potential for adverse effects of high intakes of supplemental chromium (III) and advised caution (3).

Most of the concerns regarding the long-term safety of chromium (III) supplementation arise from several studies in cell culture, suggesting chromium (III), especially in the form of chromium picolinate, may increase DNA damage (21-23). Presently, there is no evidence that chromium (III) increases DNA damage in living organisms (3), and a study in 10 women taking 400 mcg/day of chromium as chromium picolinate found no evidence of increased oxidative damage to DNA as measured by antibodies to an oxidized DNA base (24).

Several studies have demonstrated the safety of daily doses of up to 1,000 mcg of chromium for several months (16, 25). However, there have been a few isolated reports of serious adverse reactions to chromium picolinate. Kidney failure was reported five months after a six-week course of 600 mcg of chromium/day in the form of chromium picolinate (26), while kidney failure and impaired liver function were reported after the use of 1,200-2,400 mcg/day of chromium in the form of chromium picolinate over a period of four to five months (27). Individuals with pre-existing kidney or liver disease may be at increased risk of adverse effects and should limit supplemental chromium intake (3).

Copper

Toxicity

Copper toxicity is rare in the general population. Acute copper poisoning has occurred through the contamination of beverages by storage in copper containing containers as well as from contaminated water supplies (31). In the U.S., the health-based guideline for a maximum water copper concentration of 1.3

mg/liter is enforced by the Environmental Protection Agency (EPA) (32). Symptoms of acute copper toxicity include abdominal pain, nausea, vomiting, and diarrhea, which help prevent additional ingestion and absorption of copper. More serious signs of acute copper toxicity include severe liver damage, kidney failure, coma, and death. Of more concern from a nutritional standpoint is the possibility of liver damage resulting from long-term exposure to lower doses of copper. In generally healthy individuals, doses of up to 10,000 mcg (10 mg) daily have not resulted in liver damage. For this reason, the U.S. Food and Nutrition Board (FNB) recently set the tolerable upper level of intake (UL) for copper at 10 mg/day from food and supplements (5). It should be noted that individuals with genetic disorders affecting copper metabolism (Wilson's disease, Indian childhood cirrhosis, and idiopathic copper toxicosis) may be at risk of adverse effects of chronic copper toxicity at significantly lower intake levels

Iron

Toxicity
Overdose: Accidental overdose of iron-containing products is the single largest cause of poisoning fatalities in children under 6 years of age. Although the oral lethal dose of elemental iron is approximately 200-250 mg/kg of body weight, considerably less has been fatal. Symptoms of acute toxicity may occur with iron doses of 20-60 mg/kg of body weight. Iron overdose is an emergency situation because the severity of iron toxicity is related to the amount of elemental iron absorbed. Acute iron poisoning produces symptoms in four stages: 1) Within 1-6 hours of ingestion, symptoms may include nausea, vomiting, abdominal pain, tarry stools, lethargy, weak and rapid pulse, low blood pressure, fever, difficulty breathing, and coma. 2) If not immediately fatal, symptoms may subside for about 24 hours. 3) Symptoms may return 12 to 48 hours after iron ingestion and may include serious signs of failure in the following organ systems: cardiovascular, kidney, liver, hematologic (blood), and central nervous systems. 4) Long-term damage to the central nervous system, liver (cirrhosis), and stomach may develop 2 to 6 weeks after ingestion (11, 23).

Magnesium

Toxicity
Adverse effects have not been identified from magnesium occurring naturally in food. However, adverse effects from excess magnesium have been observed with intakes of various magnesium salts (supplemental magnesium). The initial symptom of excess magnesium supplementation is diarrhea—a well-known side

effect of magnesium that is used therapeutically as a laxative. Individuals with impaired kidney function are at higher risk for adverse effects from magnesium supplementation, and symptoms of magnesium toxicity have occurred in people with impaired kidney function taking moderate doses of magnesium-containing laxatives or antacids. Elevated serum levels of magnesium (hypermagnesemia) may result in a fall in blood pressure (hypotension). Some of the later effects of magnesium toxicity, such as lethargy, confusion, disturbances in normal cardiac rhythm, and deterioration of kidney function, are related to severe hypotension. As hypermagnesemia progresses, muscle weakness and difficulty breathing may occur. Severe hypermagnesemia may result in cardiac arrest (2, 4). The Food and Nutrition Board (FNB) of the Institute of Medicine set the tolerable upper level (UL) for supplemental magnesium intake in generally healthy adolescents and adults at 350 mg/day. This UL represents the highest level of daily supplemental magnesium intake likely to pose no risk of diarrhea or gastrointestinal disturbance in almost all individuals. The FNB cautions that individuals with renal impairment are at higher risk of adverse effects from excess supplemental magnesium intake. However, the FNB also notes that there are some conditions, which may warrant higher doses of magnesium under medical supervision (4).

Manganese

Toxicity

Inhaled manganese: Manganese toxicity may result in multiple neurologic problems and is a well-recognized health hazard for people who inhale manganese dust (1,4). Unlike ingested manganese, inhaled manganese is transported directly to the brain before it can be metabolized in the liver (23). The symptoms of manganese toxicity generally appear slowly over a period of months to years. In its worst form, manganese toxicity can result in a permanent neurological disorder with symptoms similar to those of Parkinson's disease, including tremors, difficulty walking, and facial muscle spasms. This syndrome is sometimes preceded by psychiatric symptoms, such as irritability, aggressiveness, and even hallucinations (24).

Methylcyclopentadienyl manganese tricarbonyl (MMT): MMT is a manganese-containing compound used in gasoline as an anti-knock additive. Although it has been used for this purpose in Canada for more than 20 years, uncertainty about adverse health effects from inhaled exhaust emissions kept the U.S. Environmental Protection Agency (EPA) from approving its use in unleaded gasoline. In 1995, a U.S. court decision made MMT available for widespread use in unleaded gasoline (23). A recent study in Montreal, where MMT had been used for more than 10 years, found airborne manganese levels to be similar to those in areas where MMT was not used (25). However, the impact of long-term exposure to low levels of MMT combustion products has not been thoroughly evaluated and will require additional study (26).

Ingested manganese: Limited evidence suggests that high manganese intakes from drinking water may be associated with neurological symptoms similar to those of Parkinson's disease. Severe neurological symptoms were reported in 25 people who drank water contaminated with manganese and probably other contaminants from dry cell batteries for 2-3 months (27). Water manganese levels were found to be 14 mg/liter almost 2 months after symptoms began and may have already been declining (1). A study of older adults in Greece found a high prevalence of neurological symptoms in those exposed to water manganese levels of 1.8-2.3 mg/liter (28), while a study of people in Germany drinking water with manganese levels ranging from 0.3-2.2 mg/liter found no evidence of increased neurological symptoms compared to those drinking water containing less than 0.05 mg/liter (29). Manganese in drinking water may be more bioavailable than manganese in food. However, none of the studies measured dietary manganese, so total manganese intake in these cases is unknown (1,4). In the U.S., the EPA recommends 0.05 mg/liter as the maximum allowable manganese concentration in drinking water (30).

A single case of manganese toxicity was reported in a person who took large amounts of mineral supplements for years (31), while another case was reported as a result of taking a Chinese herbal supplement (24). Manganese toxicity resulting from foods alone has not been reported in humans, even though certain vegetarian diets could provide up 20 mg/day of manganese (4,31).

Individuals with increased susceptibility to manganese toxicity

Chronic liver disease: Manganese is eliminated from the body mainly in bile. Thus, impaired liver function may lead to decreased manganese excretion. Manganese accumulation in individuals with cirrhosis or liver failure may contribute to neurological problems and Parkinson's disease-like symptoms (1,22).

Newborns: The newborn brain may be more susceptible to manganese toxicity due to a greater expression of receptors for the manganese transport protein (transferrin) in developing nerve cells and the immaturity of the liver's bile elimination system (4).

Due to the severe implications of manganese neurotoxicity the Food and Nutrition Board (FNB) of the Institute of Medicine set very conservative upper levels of intake (UL) for manganese, which are listed in the table below (4).

Molydenum

Toxicity

The toxicity of molybdenum compounds appears to be relatively low in humans. Increased blood uric acid levels and gout-like symptoms have been reported in occupationally exposed workers in a copper-molybdenum plant and an Armenian population consuming 10 to 15 milligrams (mg) of molybdenum from food daily (13). In other studies, blood and urinary uric acid levels were not elevated by molybdenum intakes of up to 1.5 mg/day (2). There is one report of an acute toxic reaction associated with molybdenum from a dietary supplement. An adult male, reported to have consumed a total of 13.5 mg of molybdenum over a period of 18 days (300-800 mcg/day), developed acute psychosis with hallucinations, seizures, and other neurologic symptoms (12). However, a controlled study found no serious adverse effects of molybdenum intakes of up to 1.5 mg/day (1,500 mcg/day) for 24 days in four healthy young men (9).

The Food and Nutrition Board (FNB) of the Institute of Medicine found little evidence that molybdenum excess was associated with adverse health outcomes in generally healthy people. To determine the tolerable upper level of intake, the FNB selected adverse reproductive effects in rats as the most sensitive index of toxicity and applied a large uncertainty factor because animal data was used (2). Tolerable upper intake levels (UL) for molybdenum are listed by age group in the table below.

Potassium

Toxicity (excess)

Abnormally elevated serum potassium concentrations are referred to as hyperkalemia. Hyperkalemia occurrs when potassium intake exceeds the capacity of the kidneys to eliminate it. Acute or chronic renal (kidney) failure, the use of potassium-sparing diuretics, and insufficient aldosterone secretion (hypoaldosteronism) may result in the accumulation of excess potassium due to decreased urinary potassium excretion. Oral doses greater than 18 grams taken at one time in individuals not accustomed to high intakes may lead to severe hyperkalemia, even in those with normal kidney function (4). Hyperkalemia may also result from a shift of intracellular potassium into the circulation, which may occur with the rupture of red blood cells (hemolysis) or tissue damage (e.g., trauma or severe burns). Symptoms of hyperkalemia may include tingling of the hands and feet, muscular weakness, and temporary paralysis. The most serious complication of hyperkalemia is the development of an abnormal heart rhythm (cardiac arrhythmia), which can lead to cardiac arrest (27).

Selenium

Toxicity

Although selenium is required for health, high doses can be toxic. Acute and fatal toxicities have occurred with accidental or suicidal ingestion of gram quantities of selenium. Clinically significant selenium toxicity was reported in 13 individuals after taking supplements that contained 27.3 milligrams (27,300 mcg) per tablet due to a manufacturing error. Chronic selenium toxicity (selenosis) may occur with smaller doses of selenium over long periods of time. The most frequently reported symptoms of selenosis are hair and nail brittleness and loss. Other symptoms may include gastrointestinal disturbances, skin rashes, a garlic breath odor, fatigue, irritability, and nervous system abnormalities. In an area of China with a high prevalence of selenosis, toxic effects occurred with increasing frequency when blood selenium concentrations reached a level corresponding to an intake of 850 mcg/day. The Food and Nutrition Board (FNB) recently set the tolerable upper level (UL) for selenium at 400 mcg/day in adults based on the prevention of hair and nail brittleness and loss and early signs of chronic selenium toxicity (11). The UL of 400 mcg/day for adults (see table below) includes selenium obtained from food, which averages about 100 mcg/day for adults in the U.S., as well as selenium from supplements For more information on the data used to set the recent RDA and UL for selenium, see **The New Recommendations for Dietary Antioxidants: A Response and Position Statement by the Linus Pauling Institute** in the spring/summer 2000 issue of the Linus Pauling Institute newsletter.

Zinc

Acute toxicity

Isolated outbreaks of acute zinc toxicity have occurred as a result of the consumption of food or beverages contaminated with zinc released from galvanized containers. Signs of acute zinc toxicity are abdominal pain, diarrhea, nausea, and vomiting. Single doses of 225 to 450 mg of zinc usually induce vomiting. Milder gastrointestinal distress has been reported at doses of 50 to 150 mg/day of supplemental zinc. Metal fume fever has been reported after the inhalation of zinc oxide fumes. Profuse sweating, weakness, and rapid breathing may develop within 8 hours of zinc oxide inhalation and persist 12-24 hours after exposure is terminated (4, 5).

Adverse effects

The major consequence of long-term consumption of excessive zinc is copper deficiency. Total zinc intakes of 60 mg/day (50 mg supplemental and 10 mg dietary zinc) have been found to result in signs of copper deficiency. In order to prevent copper deficiency, the U.S. Food and Nutrition Board set the tolerable upper level of intake (UL) for adults at 40 mg/day, including dietary and supplemental zinc (4).

Intranasal zinc is known to cause a loss of the sense of smell (anosmia) in laboratory animals (55), and there have been several case reports of individuals who developed anosmia after using intranasal zinc gluconate (39,40). Since zinc-associated anosmia may be irreversible, zinc nasal gels and nasal sprays should be avoided.[206]

---

[206] http://lpi.oregonstate.edu/infocenter/minerals/iron/index.html

Section 5

CONCLUSION

CHAPTER 35

The Bipolar Theory

Explanation and therapy

The very simplest explanation for bipolar disease is there is an energy leak in the body. The human body's energy is directly related to phosphate levels. In the human body phosphate is energy. I believe that only one kidney may be affected. The result of one good kidney and one diseased kidney is that the parathyroid gland is constantly making corrections for the loss of calcium and phosphate.

Imagine two people, one is normal and the other has bipolar disease. Each person begins with the same amount of energy. The normal person, all factors the same, will maintain the same energy levels over a specific length of time. Let's call the length of time a month. In the bipolar person, the energy level will decline slowly over the month because of this energy leak. For example purposes, let's call this leak amount 1 percent. As the month progesses, the bipolar person's energy level declines according to this example by 30 percent. At the end of this month the normal person is still functioning on 100 percent energy, however, the bipolar person's energy level is only 70 percent of the normal person's energy.

As the level of phosphate declines, the level of the energy compound glucose 6-phophate also declines. This compound is composed of the sugar glucose and the energy ion phosphate. It appears that the craving for sweets is tied to levels of this ion. When the levels of glucose 6-phosphate are low, then the craving for sweets is strong. (There is a genetic link between glucose 6-phosphate deficiency and bipolar disease. This theory explains this link). Remember this disease is also known as nephrogenic diabetes. A conservative to approach to sugar and carbohydrate consumption is very wise. Unfortunately, when too little phosphate is available and when the excess consumption of sugar occurs, then the body is overloaded with sugar, glucose. The body does not know that is has too much glucose because it uses glucose 6-phosphate as the marker for energy levels and hunger. What happens is the body begins making it's own glucose by using up fat and muscle through a process known as glycolysis. This results in weight loss.

The loss of protein from muscle results in increased amounts of a substance known as glutamate. This substance has been linked to attention deficits.

This may be what is happening to a person you would describe as exceptionally skinny. This excess glucose also produces a medical condition known as lactic acidosis, which produces metabolic acidosis. Acidosis, as you recall, is just too many acidic hydrogen ions floating around in the body. Glucose is a very simple compound. Glucose only contains three ions: carbon, oxygen, and hydrogen. When glucose is metabolized by the body one of the products is carbon dioxide. Therefore, there is too much carbon dioxide and acidic hydrogen ion in the body.

The body has an efficient method to remove excess carbon dioxide. The organ used is the lungs and the method is called respiration. Carbon dioxide is the stuff we exhale during breathing. In order to compensate for excess carbon dioxide due to this sugar load, the body speeds up respiration. This process is known in medical terms as respiratory alkalosis. However, there are still excess acidic hydrogen ions in the body. The body does not have an efficient method to neutralize or eliminate the excess acidic hydrogen ions because it has loss a significant quantity of its buffer or hydrogen ion acceptor, phosphate. The result in a bipolar person's case is warm skin.

The organs of the body sacrifice or down-regulate to compensate for this deficiency. The result, in this case, is the body decreases protein synthesis and bile secretion from the gall bladder. This decreased protein synthesis protects the body from deficiencies in "available" minerals. Please recall that these minerals are absolutely necessary to produce important chemicals required for the body to function. Many of these minerals are protein bound. This means they are stored on protein. Surmising, there would be too much stored away and not enough ready for use. The result would be that these minerals would be bound to proteins and, therefore, unavailable for use in catalyzing enzymes necessary for biological functions. Therefore, sacrificing or down-regulating protein synthesis is important so that the body can approach necessary levels of needed minerals to run the body's physiological processes.

Unfortunately, the loss of phosphate also down-regulates the gall bladder. This results in decreased absorption, storage, and possibly increased excretion of necessary minerals that are involved with the bile system. These minerals are very important in the production or synthesis of many chemicals in the nervous system. The result is that biological functions such as sleep, mood, filtering thoughts (needed to prevent that feeling of being overwhelmed), and others are affected.

At this point the body's regulatory calcium and phosphate system, the parathyroid gland, calculates that the bipolar person's energy level is critically low. In this case, the body responds by directly reabsorbing the energy ion phosphate, probably through extrarenal vitamin D3 synthesis. (See my blood work). Please recall that active vitamin D3 helps in the absorption and reabsorption of the energy ion phosphate. This would help restore energy. The trouble is that the body may overshoot. This would result in hypomania.

This synthesis of extrarenal vitamin D3 may be stimulated by cortisol. (See blood work). Therefore, in this scenario we see this person's energy level rise rapidly. For a short while, this person will feel renewed and energized. However, this "jump start" or hypomania, comes at a price. Cortisol and steroids, in general, decrease immunity. It may be that cortisol acts on the bones to increase synthesis of extrarenal vitamin D3 and to acquire phosphate from the bone. This increases phosphate levels. However, this person may get a cold because he cannot fight off infection. Because the body cannot sustain improved energy levels depression may result. Other factors may be involved with immunitiy as well, because zinc and vitamin C are also vitallly linked to immunity.

Mineral levels determine whether a person has hypomania, mania, or psychosis. Severely deficient mineral levels result in severely altered production of nervous system chemicals, neurotransmitters. Some minerals, like magnesium, act as a guard at nervous system gateways to slow the rate of nervous system activity. When this guard is away, mineral deficiency, there is a stampede of nervous system activity. When deficiencies in minerals like copper occur, which are involved in the production of the substance melatonin (required for sleep), then insomnia results. I have read that with severe sleep deprivation a subtance similar to LSD is manufactered in the brain. Obviously, this can have bizaare consequences.

The ion phosphate is very important in buffering the body. This means phosphate neutralizes excess acid in the body. It is very effective at buffering because has the ability to accept three acidic hydrogen ions for every available phosphate ion. A poor substitute, chloride ion, is reabsorbed due to this deficiency. Chloride ion can only accept one acidic hydrogen ion for each available chloride ion. The result is a much larger quantity of chloride ion being reabsorbed. This causes many side effects like anxiety and apprehension. A person deficient in the gatekeeper, magnesium ion, will have a stampede of chloride ion entering the nervous system. This excessive reabsorption of chloride may also result in alkaline urine. This may cause urinary tract problems.

Therefore, in this condition we see both respiratory alkalosis and metabolic acidosis. We also see hypoparathyroidism and hyperparathyroidism. It is no wonder that this condition has never been described in physical terms before because it is like a mirror looking at its reflection.

How is stress involved? Stress has the ability to inhibit production of the active vitamin D. This results in the loss of the energy ion, phosphate. Therefore, stress "revs-up" this disorder with disastrous consequences. Everything in this sequence would be stronger and faster. This means that a larger quantity of chloride ion would be reabsorbed at a faster rate and the volume of mineral loss would be much, much larger. The minerals are "bleached out" of the body. If this highly stressful situation persists for a significant length of time, then psychosis would be the expectation.

As mentioned in the first chapter, the drug calictriol, used with phosphate supplementation, may be a key to resolving most of these problems. I do not have experience with this therapy. However, I have personally benefited from calcium loading when used in conjunction with phosphate supplementation. This leads me to believe that using calcitriol will work. This would tremendously simplify this therapy, which would be good news. The quantity of calcitriol would probably differ considerably from that used by someone who has kidney failure.

In summary, bipolar disease appears to be a mild form of distal renal tubular acidosis, also known as nephrogenic diabetes. This condition occurs because of the failure to produce active vitamin D, DHCC, in the macula densa of the kidney. This is due to 1 alpha hydroxylase failure at probably the distal renal tubule and possibly the proximal renal tubule in "one or both" kidneys. This results in the failure to reabsorb phosphate ion. The enzyme 7 alpha hydroxylase also appears to be affected. The lack of this enzyme can down-regulate bile synthesis. This results in many important biological pathways being affected, particularly those involving mood and sleep. Bipolar disease is a "mild chronic condition" that results in "covert leaching" of all alkali except sodium. A bipolar person has the bare minimum of minerals required for normal function, and any stress overloads the system.

This is the therapy I use to treat my disease. It may seem somewhat cumbersome, but it works for me. People prone to kidney stones or gallstones should NOT use this therapy unless under the advice of a physician. If you attempt this program understand that your doctor is absolutely necessary to ensure your overall safety. Beware that acid-base disturbances and mineral toxicity could occur. Your doctor is in the best position to evaluate your condition. Personally, I have not experienced any side effects, especially when compared to the prescription medicines I have taken in the past, but the possibility does exist if these supplements are used excessively high doses or if other medical conditions exist. All of these items are naturally found in the body. Understand that when I say reduce that is what I mean. It does not mean exclude. In this therapy nothing in a normal diet is excluded. Items are simply reduced to achieve balance.

Dennis Miller's Bipolar Therapy

(1) <u>Reduce milk</u> (no more than 2 glasses per day) and avoid products fortified with vitamin D. Some orange juice products are fortified with vitamin D. These should be avoided. I used to drink an enormous amount of milk. I have experienced some of the toxic effects of excessive vitamin D consumption. I believe these symptoms are related to excessive consumption vitamin D fortified milk. Vitamin D is a fat-soluble vitamin; therefore, it may take a while for the symptoms of toxicity to disappear. Fat-soluble vitamins dissolve in the fat and are stored. My theory is that a very lean person may have less fat to dissolve and store this vitamin. Their metabolism of vitamin D may be significantly different from a normal person with adequate fat stores. Personally, I have noticed a disappearance of migraine symptoms; particularly right eye pain.

(2) <u>Reduce table salt.</u> Reduce products with high chloride ion content specifically table salt. This includes breads that contain high amounts of sodium chloride. My theory is that *excess chloride ion results in excitability.* (Even artificial table salt may include high levels of chloride).

(3) <u>Calcium carbonate.</u> Consume 2 or 3 tablets of <u>Tums Ultra</u> two or three times a day to stimulate the parathyroid gland to produce more 1 alpha hydroxylase; plus the carbon dioxide will help with acid-base balance. This also stimulates GI absorption of the energy ion, phosphate. Note that cola drinks contain phosphoric acid and theoretically non-cola drinks may predispose a person more to wet Beriberi like symptoms. I chew my Tums and I follow that with a half glass of <u>diet cola</u>. My energy levels have improved dramatically.

(4) <u>Sodium bicarbonate</u>. If your skin feels warm it may be necessary to use sodium bicarbonate to restore acid-base balance. Sodium bicarbonate should only be used during episodes of warm skin. Potassium bicarbonate is preferred to sodium bicarbonate, but potassium bicarbonate is a prescription item. The sodium in sodium bicarbonate may lead to high blood pressure or hypernatremia. Therefore, using sodium bicarbonate conservatively is wise. At least in my case, sodium is preferentially reabsorbed which leads to higher sodium blood levels.

(5) <u>Orange juice</u>. The potassium in orange juice helps restore levels that are lost from acidosis. Orange juice is also high in vitamin C. Orange juice contains citric acid, which is important for acid-base balance. Orange juice also serves as a vehicle. Orange juice can make the magnesium citrate very palatable. Orange juice is my friend.

(6) <u>Mineral supplementation</u>. In addition to calcium and potassium supplementation, magnesium, manganese, zinc, copper, iron, boron, cobalt, selenium are excessively excreted and supplementation is necessary. I have included a great deal of information about each item for reference purposes.

If you choose to supplement be sure to use minerals that are absorbed optimally. Magnesium supplementation is important. Remember this is important for mood and energy. I have found that between 1/2 to 1 teaspoons of magnesium citrate powder mixed in my orange juice once or twice a day is effective. Many of these products can produce toxicity if used incorrectly. Your doctor is best suited in determining your appropriate dose. One of the best food sources for minerals that I have found is cashews. Possibly somewhere along the line, a person with this disease found that cashews were effective. This may be how the term "nut" was coined. Cashews provide significant quantities of about every mineral needed, except chromium. Generally, though, a little chromium goes a long way. An excellent food source of chromium is beets.

(7) <u>Iron.</u> Iron supplementation that includes vitamin C may help the kidney produce more 1-alpha hydroxylase. You doctor should evaluate iron supplementation. Excessive intake is possibly dangerous. Generally speaking bipolar people will have low iron levels and, therefore, supplementation would be recommended. I recommend a 30-minute walk in the morning at least three times a week for UV exposure to stimulate natural vitamin D production. I do not know if there are any metabolically differences between naturally produced vitamin D and vitamin D supplements. Hopefully, our medical researchers will be able to provide this answer. It is important for a person using this therapy to know the symptoms of vitamin D toxicity. (In my case I have mild right eye pain when levels of vitamin D have been exceeded.)

(8) <u>Avoid stress</u>. An understanding of the symptoms and effects that stress can produce is important. Orange urine, excessive carbohydrate consumption, or sweaty palms may identify stress. I have found that folic acid and vitamin B-12 are valuable in combating stress. The form of vitamin B-12 that is dissolved under the tongue is more effective that the oral preparation. I have not evaluated any of the ubiquitous stress relief programs available in the bookstores, but I may do so in the future. One seminar I went to a few years ago as part of my continuing education stated that just having <u>someone to listen to your problems without them making judgments</u> generally brings about stress relief. Your minister may be very helpful in this regard.

(9) <u>Be aware of increases in carbohydrate or alcohol consumption.</u> This may be a sign that something significant needs to be corrected. It is not unusual for a person with this disease to eat a half-gallon of ice cream. Ice cream is high in calcium and carbohydrate. *Thiamine requirement is proportional to caloric intake.*[207] A person using this therapy should choose protein as a snack instead of sweets. This is because protein produces slow and steady glucose levels; not the quick high and free-falling lows of sugar. A person with bipolar disease according to my theory will be expected to have low calcium levels. Stress can produce significant calcium losses. These losses produce calcium craving. The result is an ice cream binge. A strong craving for carbohydrate may signal a decline in glucose 6-phosphate. Remember this is the body's energy compound. This may be the appropriate time to take Tums, drink diet cola and eat a protein snack. A diabetic type of approach to diet is helpful. Therefore, avoid all beverage that contain high fructose corn syrup. An important point to recall is that alcohol is a carbohydrate. This "snack" may help prevent you from "needing a drink."

The same could be said for alcohol probably. Alcohol is an alternate carbohydrate source. Alcohol does, however, free magnesium and possibly other protein bound ions. This would temporarily make a person with this disease feel better, but the effect would be short term and the person would excrete those ions. The result is you feel worse later. Remember this disease is also known as neprogenic diabetes. A conservative approach toward sugar and carbohydrate consumption is warranted. This disease creates strong carbohydrate cravings due to glucose 6-phosphate deficiency. A high carbohydrate diet in a bipolar person is a diet of destruction.

It is important for people with bipolar disease to choose foods with a low glycemic index. Rick Mendosa at provides a list of foods: http://www.stanford.edu/~dep/gilists.htm.

(10) A <u>high potency vitamin B complex with C</u> that does not contain vitamin D is very, very valuable, but note that additional folic acid may be necessary because of government the maximum dose is 0.4 mg over the counter. The vitamin B complex and C supplement I use is Z-Bec. The government's reason is because folic acid may hide a disease known as pernicious anemia. Your doctor is adequately suited to make a recommendation of your folic acid need. Because vitamin B's and C are water-soluble they are not stored in the

---

[207] Harrison's Principles of Internal Medicine, 10th Edition.

body like the fat-soluble vitamin A, D, and E, therefore, it is necessary to take water-soluble vitamins more than once a day.

Because vitamin B12 may not be absorbed properly an over the counter preparation that allows dissolution under the tongue is preferable. A prescription injectable preparation is available through your doctor.

(11) <u>Copper and thiamine</u>. At bedtime, I take an absorbable copper supplement and thiamine. These two items stimulate melatonin production necessary for sleep. If you are still having problems sleeping about ¼ tablet of melatonin may help induce sleep.

(12) <u>Avoid caffeine.</u> Excessive consumption of caffeine may lead to insomnia. This is especially true if the body's stores of the mineral molybdenum are deficient. If there is a molydenum deficiency, then caffeine may not be metabolized efficiently. The result is a little caffeine will go a very long way.

My short list would read: Tums, diet cola, Z-Bec, cashews, and a capsule of absorbable copper at bedtime to induce sleep. It is also important to <u>know the physical complaints</u>, see table 1, and learn the mineral deficiency associated with that complaint.

It may be that a high phosphate diet with calcitriol may help this condition, but I do not have experience with this therapy. *Vitamin D-resistant, familial and nonfamilial, hyposphosphatemic rickets are treated with inorganic phosphate and calcitriol.*[208] For some of us, that is the bipolar community, **supplementation with active 1,25 DHCC, also known as calcitriol, may be sufficient for restoring health.** It must be noted that some people with rickets do not respond to this drug. In additional, for those of us in the bipolar community that have *only one kidney affected* the effectiveness of this drug is questionable and up for investigative studies.

It is important for athletes to understand the limits that bipolar disease places on their bodies. This does not mean they should stop their athletic activity, but that it is more important to have an even better understanding of bipolar disease because of the extreme dehydration and mineral losses associated with this activity. Supplementation in this case is absolutely necessary.

Getting fresh air on a regular basis will help the metabolism to keep the body running at optimum efficiency. I recommend a brisk 10 or 20-minute walk in the morning at least three times a week.

---

[208] Merck Manual, 15th Edition, page 974

URO-BILIARY PSYCHOSIS PATHWAY

1 alpha hydroxylase failure in kidney
◆
Active vitamin D failure; 1,25 dihydroxycholecalciferol
◆
Low phosphate levels, hypophosphatemia
◆
Sweet craving stimulated
◆
Glycolysis stimulated
◆
Attention deficits

Bicarbonate reabsorption fails, excess chloride ion reabsorbed.

7 alpha hydroxylase down-regulates bile metabolism resulting in mineral losses of copper and manganese	Hyperchloremic metabolic acidosis increases urinary excretion of calcium, magnesium, zinc, cobalt and iron

Stress stimulates cortisol synthesis

Cortisol inhibits active vitamin D synthesis

Increased mineral losses with excess chloride ion

PSYCHOSIS

URO-BILIARY MINERAL LOSSES

URINARY MINERALS	ENZYME	RESULT	SYMPTOM
Zinc deficiency	↓ Anhydrase	Acid-Base imbalance	Warm skin
Potassium deficiency		Hypokalemia	Cramping and tiredness
Magnesium deficiency	ATP-ase pump failure	Metabolism slows	Constipation
Magnesium deficiency	Calcium channel blocking failure	Glutamate excitation	Attention deficits
Magnesium deficiency	Alpha ketoglutamine	GABA deficiency	Mood
Magnesium deficiency	Acetylcholine	ADH deficiency	↑ Urination and dilated eyes
URINARY MINERALS	ENZYME	RESULT	SYMPTOM
Calcium deficiency		Parathyroid aberrations	Skeletal defects
Iron deficiency		Anemia	Tiredness
Iron deficiency	↓ Melatonin transferase	↓ Melatonin	Insomnia
Chromium deficiency	↓ Glucose tolerance factor	↓ Glucose tolerance	Diabetes-like syndrome
BILE MINERALS	ENZYME	RESULT	SYMPTOM
Copper deficiency	↓ Tyrosine hydroxylase	Dopamine deficiency	Tremor, overwhelmed
Copper deficiency	↓ Tryptophan hydroxylase	Melatonin deficiency	Insomnia
Manganese deficiency		↓ Vitamin K	Increased bleeding time
Manganese deficiency	Alpha ketoglutamine	GABA deficiency	Mood
Cobalt deficiency	↓ Vitamin B-12	↑ Homocyteine	Nervous system affected

CHAPTER 36

Early dectection

Hope for the future

Nothing in this book suggests that a person should avoid medical profession-als. It is my hope that this book will advance the knowledge of this disease in order to enable the patient and the medical professional to come to a better method of therapy. I believe there is a place for prescription drugs during episodes of stress or depression. However, I also believe that the majority of prob-lems associated with this disease can be treated with the therapy I have outlined.

I am a father. Because I am a father, I care for my loved ones. I have spent most of the past year researching this condition. When my son was sick and the medi-cine was not working, I knew I had to act. If I was told a year ago that I would be completing a book the next year I would have thought that person to be "touched." I would research a topic and I would then take a chance on experi-mentation. Each experiment provided exciting results. At no time during this research did I come to a roadblock. I absolutely expected a roadblock. For me this has been a scientific and spiritual exploration. Spiritual people call it a calling. I believe this was my calling. I think I have come up with a convincing explanation for bipolar disease. The people that have this disease lead lives of perpetual tor-ment. Society rarely acts with understanding or sympathy for people with this condition. Consequently, taking one's life becomes a logical means to eliminate the pain. Hopefully, this therapy will excuse those of us with this condition from the death sentence we inherited at birth. I feel certain that if programs were insti-tuted for *early childhood detection* that this disease can be identified and treated. I believe these children can and will grow up to lead absolutely normal lives. I believe these children can enjoy a life that the rest of society takes for granted.

Nothing in this book suggests that a person should avoid medical profes-sionals. The physician is a necessity. It is my hope that this book will advance the knowledge of this disease in order to enable the patient and the medical professional to come to a better method of therapy. I also believe there is a place for prescription drugs during episodes of stress or depression. However, I also believe that the majority of problems associated with this disease can be treated with the therapy I have outlined. The economic impact could possibly be enormous especially in increased productivity. However, the social impact may be more important.

The information in this book should not mislead people into believing that all the problems with bipolar condition are solved. There will probably be psychosocial issues of considerable relevance that will need to be addressed as well.

This disease I believe is much like menopause. In both conditions calcium and phosphate are affected. In both conditions emotional responsiveness is heightened. **Bipolar disease, however, is like having menopause for a lifetime.** All of you know the old expression "lift yourself up by the bootstraps." In this disease you don't even have the boots because your energy is constantly being depleted. Every time you get out a match to light the grill remember that the match is a phosphorous compound. It is phosphorous that provides the spark in your life. "Normal" people do not realize how easy they have it. The closest I have ever consistently come to normal is with this therapy. The life I have now is easy when compared to my pre-bipolar theory days. I have not had a full year on this program, yet I believe whole-heartedly in this theory. My physician has recognized my improvement. He recommends that I continue with my therapy. However, minor problems may occur. Please take your doctor a copy of this book. Once he reads and understands this book, then he can make the determination of what is best for you.

It is my greatest hope that this disease can in the near future be detected and treated at a very early stage in development so that the body and mind can develop properly. I hope that the medical community sincerely considers this evidence. If they do, I am sure they will come to the same conclusion I have. Once that acceptance occurs, then early detection and treatment will certainly follow.

This book should be used in coordination with your doctor in the hope that better therapy will be the outcome. It is important to recognize that you should not do this alone. Like with most things inappropriate use can have significant consequences. Human physiology relies on balance and your physician is in the best position to help your achieve the vitamin and mineral balance required for success in this therapy.

You ask, "How is my son?" I wish you could see his broad smile, the twinkle in his eyes, and the sound of his laughter. I am a happy father.

EPILOGUE

In the polar extremes of life experience, I once thought that being shackled was the absolute low point of my life. However, the sight of my son in shackles has replaced that low. No crime had been committed. This was done for our protection, I understand.

As a young man I could never have written a book with this considerable potential for embarrassment, but now I do so with intent and purpose. My many experiences with this disease have given me many lessons in humility. However, I had to put aside those feelings for the good of the whole. I simply want to do whatever I can to prevent others from the torment and pain of my life's bad experiences. In a way these experiences are symbolic. We, as society, may now have the ability to free people with bipolar disease from the chains that bind them.

It has been a year since that fateful night. This year has involved the stress of incredible lows, but now considerable hope prevails. This hope is not only for me, but also for the other fathers that are faced with the incredibly horrible consequences of this disease. I have cited over 200 footnotes. I intentionally stayed away from questionable or dubious sources. I cited undisputed reputable sources like the National Institute of Health, major universities, and medical texts. The point is that by using unassailable sources the plausibility of this theory becomes undeniable. In other words, it must be considered.

As a pharmacist, I come into contact with an enormous variety of people. Their illnesses or maladies are numerous. An unusual conversation occurred at work one night. I spoke with a lady that I had become familiar because her husband had been badly burned in an industrial accident. I noticed that he was seeing a psychiatrist. His doctor was now prescribing him "lithium carbonate". The question that came to my mind was, "Why is this man being treated for bipolar disease?" This is, by all accounts, a hereditary disorder, not an acquired disorder. The answer, I concluded, was that he was losing excessive amounts of valuable minerals through the extensive skin lesions. I want to thank you Mike. You did not know it, but your accident played a valuable part in establishing my hypothesis.

I chose the "Salts of the Earth" portion of the title because it relates well with context of the manuscript. That is, we are talking about minerals and minerals can be in salt form. I also chose this portion of the title because I know society, in general, excludes a bipolar person from consideration as "the salt of the earth". The other portion of the title, "Synthetic Insanity," I chose because the medicine mentioned produces a condition similar to bipolar disease. I also chose this portion of the title because the words tend to interest the reader. This interest hopefully will result in sales. Some people may look at that statement with a jaded eye. I, however, think this is a good thing because more sales mean more readers. More readers mean the message is spreading. This is absolutely a good thing.

I want to make myself available to the community by providing my email address, which is: dennisrants@yahoo.com. My sons and I intend to develop a Website to answer the most common questions and concerns. The events of my life have led me in a different direction. This direction I intend to follow until success or failure. No one is more surprised by the completion of this book than I. As I said before, I am not working in the field of academics. I began with a very basic premise. "What am I seeing?" The answer was "body heat." Every event, footnote, pathway, and theory led from that single question. After over 140 pages, 200 footnotes, and 10 months publication is ready. If this book only helps one child, teenager, or college student from the ultimate act, then my time has been well spent.

Selected Reading

Harrison's Principles of Internal Medicine, 10th Edition, 1983.
Pages used in preparation include: 118-124, 182-184, 220-236, 309, 430-431, 455-456, 461-472, 490-495, 512-513, 536, 542-543, 574-575, 587-616, 637-657, 679-686, 740, 1518, 1697, 1928-1948, 2112-2132.

The Merck Manual, 15th Edition, 1987.
Pages used in preparation include: 894-1015, 1017-1090, 2485.

The Bipolar Child: The Definitive and Reassuring Guide to Childhood's Most Misunderstood Disorder, by Demitri Papolos and Janice Papolos.

Call Me Anna: The Autobiography of Patty Duke, by Patty Duke.

BIBLIOGRAPHY

Amino Acid Transmitters [Internet], 204-522B Unit 7. Available from:
http://www.psych.mcgill.ca/courses/522/UNIT7.htm

Jeffrey L. Arnold, MD, Hypophoshatemia [Internet], eMedicine.com. June 29,
2001. Available from: http://www.emedicine.com/emerg/topic278.htm

Noriko Ashizawa, Rei Fjuimura, Kumpei Tokuyama, and Masashige Suzuki, A
bout of resistance exericse increases urinary calcium independently of osteoclastic activation in men [Internet].Journal of Applied Physiology; Vol. 83, No.
4, 1997. Available from: http://jap.physiology.org/cgi/content/full/83/4/1159

Bipolar World [Internet]. Colleen Sullivan. 2004. Available from:
http://www.bipolarworld.net/Diagnosis/Diagnosis/mania.html

Bonilla E, Salazar E, Villasmil JJ, Villalobos R, The regional distribution of
manganese in the normal brain [Internet]. National Library of Medicine,
Neurochemistry, Feb. 1982, Vol. 7, Issue 2, pp 221-227. Available from:
http://www.ncbi.nlm.nih.gov/PubMed/

Virginia A. Boundy, Stephen J. Gold, Chad J. Messer, Jingshan Chen, Jin H.
Son, Tong H. Joh, and Eric Nesterl, Regulation of Tyrosine Hydroxylase
Promoter Activity by Chronic Morphine ni TH9.0LacZ Transgenic Mice
[Internet], The Journal of Neuroscience,Vol. 18, Issue 23, pp 9989-9995.
Available from: http://www.jneurosci.org/cgi/content/full/18/23/9989

F. H. Bradley, Epilepsy and Nutritional Supplementation [Internet], November
22, 1997.
http://neuro-www.mgh.harvard.edu/forum/EpilepsyF/
11.22.973.29AMEpilepsyNutritio

Beth Carlsen, Nutrition Digest [Internet], Enerex Botanical, Ltd. 2001.
Available from: http://www.enerex.ca/nutrition_digest_book.htm#Bb11

Jeffrey D. Carron, MD, Parathryoid Physiology [Internet], July10, 2002. Available from: http://www.emedicine.com/ent/topic539.htm

Christoper J. Cooksey, Peter J. Garratt, Edward J. Land, Christopher A. Ramsden, and Patrick A Riley, Tyrosinase kinetics: failure of the auto-activation mechanism of monohydric phenol oxidation by rapid formation of a quinomethane intermediate;Great Britain, Biochemistry Journal, Volume 333, 1998, pages 685-691. Available from: http://www.biochemj.org/bj/333/0685/3330685.pdf

Tamer Coskun, Heidi K. Baumgartner, Shaoyou Chu, and Marshal H. Montrose. Coordinated regulation of gastric chloride secretion with both acid and alkali secretion [Internet]. American Journal of Physiology-Gastrointestinal and Liver Physiology, Vol. 283, Issue 5, G1147-1155, November 2002. Available from: http://ajpgi.physiology.org/cgi/content/full/283/5/G1147

Yvette Cruz, MD, Bipolar Affective Disorder. [Internet] Department of Psychiatry, Pennsylvania Medical Center, Philadelphia, Pa: Review 6.2.2002. Available from: http://www.swmedicalcenter.com/13003.cfm

L.J. Deftos, MD. Calcium and Phosphate Homeostasis, Chapter 2 [Internet]; April 2002. LI. Available from: http://www.endotext.com

Endocrine Control of Calcium and Phophate Homeostasis [Internet]. Colorado State University, October 2003. Available from: http://arblcvmbs.colostate.edu/hbooks/pathphysendocrine/thyroid/calcium.html

Endocrineweb.com, Hypoparathryoidism. Available from: http://endocrineweb.com/0_old/hypopara.html

Murray Epstein, MD, Alchols Impact on Kidney Function [Internet], Volume 21, No. 1, 1997. Available from: http://www.niaaa.nih.gov/publications/arh21-1/84.pdf

ExPASy Molecular Biology Server (Roche Biochemical Pathways) [Internet]. Available from: http://kr.expasy.org/

Expert Group on Vitamins and Minerals, Review of Cobalt [Internet], EVM/00/07/P. Available from: http://archive.food.gov.uk/committees/evm/papers/evm7.pdf

John L. Farber, Mechanisms of Cell Injury by Activated Oxygen Species [Internet], eph online, Department of Pathology, Jefferson Medical College, Thomas Jefferson University, Philadelphia, PA. Available from: http://ehis.niehs.nih/members/1994/Suppl-10/farber-full.html

Mark Goodarzi, MD, UCLA Endocrinology, Hypercalcemia [Internet]. Available from: http://www.endocrinology.med.ucla.edu/hypercalcemia.htm

Gpnotebook, Copper deficiency, Oxbridge Solution, Ltd, 2003. Available from: http://www.gpnotebook.co.uk/cache/-50292321.htm

Dr. G. Gray, Amino Acid Degradation and the Urea Cycle[Internet]. Southwest Baptist University. Available from: http://www.sbuniv.edu/~ggray.wh.bol/CHE3364/b1c25out.htm

Harrison's Principles of Internal Medicine, 10th Edition, (NY: McGraw-Hill, 1983).
Pages used in preparation include: 118-124, 182-184, 220-236, 309, 430-431, 455-456, 461-472, 490-495, 512-513, 536, 542-543, 574-575, 587-616, 637-657, 679-686, 740, 1518, 1697, 1928-1948, 2112-2132.

Hypechloremic Acidosis [Internet], 1998. Available from: http://anaesthetist.com/icu/elec/nagacid.htm

Johns Hopkins Pathology, Gallbladder and Bile Duct Cancer [Internet], July 2001. Available from: http://pathology2.jhu.edu/bileduct/anataphys.cfm

Noriatu Kanno, Gene LeSage, Shannon Glaser, and Gianfranco Alpini. Regulation of cholangiocyte bicarbonate secretion [Internet]. American Journal of Physiology-Gastrointestinal and Liver Physiology, Vol 281, Issue 3, G612-G625, September 2001. Available from: http://ajpgi.physiology.org/cgi/content/full/283/5/G1147

Kaye H. Kilburn, Brain but not lung functions impaired after a chlorine incident[Internet], Industrial Health 2003, 41, 299-305. Available from: http://www.niih.go.jp/en/indu_hel/2003/pdf/ih_41_4_01.pdf

Michael W. King, Ph. D [Internet]., August 16, 2003. Available from: http://web.indstate.edu/thcme/mwking/aminoacidderivatives.html

Michael W. King, Ph. D. Regulation of Cellular Sterol Content [Internet], IU School of Medicine; September 29, 2003. Available from: http://web.indstate.edu/thcme/mwking/cholesterol.html#bile

Michael W. King, Ph. D. Indiana University School of Medicine[Internet]; August 12, 2003. Available from: http://www.indstate.edu/thcme/mwking/vitamins.html

Shawna Kopchu, RN, Hypomagnesemia [Internet], The Barttersite. Available from: http://www.barttersite.com/hypomagnesemia.htm

Nancy F. Krebs, Overview of Zinc Absorption and Excretion in the Human Gastrointestinal Tract [Internet], Journal of Nutrition, Vol. 2000, Issue 130, pp 1374S-1377S. Available from: http://www.nutrition.org/cgi/content/full/130/5/1374S

Sean C. Kumer,Kent E. Vrana, Intricate Regulation of Tyrosine Hydroxylay and Genese Activity Expression [Internet]. Journal of Neurochemistry, Vol 67, Issue 2, page 443, August 1996. Availabe from: http://www.blackwell-synergy.com

Eleanor Lederer, MD. Hypophosphatemia [Internet], eMedicine.com, March 28, 2003. Available from: http://www.emedicine.com/med/topic/1135.htm

Stephen W Leslie, MD, Hypercalciuria[Internet], eMedicine.com Vol. 3, No. 8, August 29, 2002. Available from: http://author.emedicine.com/MED/topic1069.htm

Linus Pauling Institute. Oregon State University [Internet]. Available from: http://www.lpi.oregonstate.edu/infocenter/minerals.html

Louisiana State University, School of Medicine in New Orleans [Internet]. Available from: http://www.physciology.lsuhsc.edu/mgl/7.asp

Rafael Luboshitzky, Pyridoxine and Melatonin Secretion[Internet], Neuroendocrinology Letters; NEL Vol 23, No 3, June 2002. Available from: http://www.nel.edu/23_3/NEL230302A02_Luboshitzky.htm

James T. McCarthy, Rajiv Kumar, Divalent Cation Metabolism: Magnesium [Internet]. Available from: http://www.kidneyatlas.org/book1/adk1_04.pdf

L. E. Mallette, K Khouri, H. Zengotita, B. W. Hollis, and S. Malini, Lithium treatment increases intact and midregion parathyroid hormone and parathyroid volume [Internet] Journal of Clinical Endocrinology & Metabolism, Vol 68, 654-660, Copyright © 1989 by Endocrine Society. Available from: http://jcem.endojournals.org/cgi/content/abstract/68/3/654

Peter J. Mallow, J. Wesley Pike, and David Feldman, The Vitamin D Receptor and the Syndrome of Hereditary 1,25 Dihydroxyvitamin D-Resistant Rickets, [Internet] Endocrine Reviews; 20 (2): 156-188 copyright 1999 by the Endocrine Society. Available from: http://edrv.endojournals.org/cgi/content/full/20/2/156

Medline Plus, Thomson MICROMEDEX, March 2004. Available from: http://www.nlm.nih.gov/medlineplus/druginfo/uspdi/202114.html

Medscape from WebMD, Breastfeeding: Unraveling the Mysteries of Mother's Milk [Internet], General Medicine; Vol. 1, Issue 1, 1999. Available from: http://www.medscape.com/content/1996/00/40/88/408813/408813_tab.html

The Merck Manual, 15th Edition. Rathway, (NJ Merck & Co., Inc. 1987). Pages used in preparation include: 894-1015, 1017-1090, 2485.

National Association of Mental Illness. Available from: http://namiwi.nami.org/helpline/teensuicide.html

National Instiute of Health, National Institute of Diabetes and Digestive and Kidney Diseases,Wilson Disease[Internet]. NIH Publication No. 03-4684, March 2003. Available from: http://digestive.niddk.nih.gov/ddiseases/pubs/wilson/index.htm

Northwestern University Medical School, 1 Nutritional Demands of Diesease and Trauma Lecture 89, 2000. Available from: http://www.nums.nwu.ed

Demitri Papolos and Janice Papolos,The Bipolar Child, Broadway Press, page 165.

Pares A, Rimola A, Bruguera M, Mas E, Rodes J., Renal tubular acidosis in primary biliary cirrhosis [Internet]; Gastroenterology, Volume 80, Issue 4, pages 681-6, April 1981. Available from: http://www.ncbI.nlm.nih.gov/entrez/

The Parietal Cell: Mechanism of Acid Secretion [Internet]. Colorado State University. Available from: http://www.vivo.colostate.edu/hbooks/pathphys/digestion/stomach/parietal.html

Emilio Petrone, Rachel Goldman, Karim Calis, George P. Chrousos, Giovanni Cizza Glucocorticoid-Induced Osteoporosis Basic Mechanisms and Clinical Implications, Chapter 5, Endotext.com [Internet]. May, 12, 2003.Available from: http://www.endotext.com/adrenal/adrenal7/adrenalframe7.htm

Physiology and Pharmaclogy: Chapter 28: : Adrenocorticosteroids/ Adrenocortical Antagonists [Internet]. Available from: http://www.pharmacology2000.com/Adrenocorticosteroids/physiol1.htm

D. Dean Potter, Jr. MD An Elderly Woman with Recurrent Hyperparathyroidism [Internet]. Dowden Health Media: Contemporary Surgery; vol. 58, no. 11, November 2002, page 555. Avaialble from: http://www.contemporarysurgery.com/11_02/1102Hypp.pdf

Klaus Radebold, MD, Achlorhydria [Internet], eMedicine Journal, Vol. 3, No. 7, July 11, 2002. Available from: http://author.emedicine.com/MED/topic18.htm

Philip Salen, MD, Hyperparathroidism [Internet]. June 28, 2001. Available from: http://www.emedicine.com/emerg/topic265.htm

Yehuda Shoenfeld, Maurizio Cutolo, The Glucocorticoid Induces Osteoporosis [Internet] International Congess, March 2003, Turin, Italy. Available from: David A. Eckerman, Ph. D [Internet]. Available from: http://www.rheuma21st.com/archives/report_gio_int_cong_shoefeld_cutolo.html

Secretion of Bile and the Role of Bile Acids in Digestion [Internet], 2001. Colorado State University. Available from: http://arbl.cvmbs.colostate.edu/hbooks.pathphys/digestion/liver/ble/html

Segawa Disease/DYT5, Dopa-Responsive dystonia [Internet].
aamm.unm.edu/get_pic.php?p_id=213

Rich Smith, Osteoporosis: The Search for a Cure[Internet], Vol 2, No. 7,
July/August 2000; Vol 3, No.4, July/Auguest 2001. Available from:
http://www.orthopedictechreview.com/issues/julaug00/page30.htm

Stress and Memory [Internet]. Available from:
http://socrates.berkeley.edu/~psy114/week14_lecture.html

Sutera, Glycolysis [Internet]. Biology News, Ecology Key Concepts; Week
5/8/2000. Sut Available from: http://www.duke.edu:~djs3bio/

The National Academy of Sciences, 1 alpha, 25 vitamin D3 regulates transcrip-
tion of of carbonic anhydrase II mRNA in avian melanocytes [Internet]. 1992.
Available from: http://www.pnas.org

The Journal of Biological Chemistry [Internet], Stanford University.Journal of
Biological Chemistry, Vol. 278, Issue 8, 5929-5940, Feb. 21, 2003 Available
from: http://www.jbc.org/content/full/278/8/5929

Trace Element Requirements and Mineral Deficiencies [Internet]. Available
from: http://surgery.mc.duke.edu/nutrition/secure/trace_elements.html

Marek Treiman, Jorgen Warberg, Endocrine Glands in Humans [Internet].
Available from: http://www.mfi.ku.dk.ppaulev/chapter30/Chapter%2030.htm

Tuula E. Tuormaa, FORESIGHT, the Association for the Promotion of
Preconceptual Care [Internet]. Journal of Orthomolecular Medicine, 11 (3):
69-79, Sept. 1996. Available from: http://www.foresight-preconception.org.uk

Tyrosinase [Internet]. PF00264. Available from:
http://pfam.wustl.edu/cgi-bin/getdesc?acc=PF00264

University of Maryland Medicine. Manganese [Internet]. April 2002. Available
from: http://www.umm.edu/altmed/ConsSupplements/Manganesecs.html

Peter Wilkes, Hypoproteinemia, strong ion difference, and acid-base status in
critically ill patients[Internet]. Journal of Applied Physiology, Vol. 84, Issue 5,
1740-1748, May 1998. Available from:
http://jap.physiology.org/cgi/content/full/84/5/1740

Danny Winder, Ph.D., Synapse III [Internet], Vanderbilt University School of Medicine, January 16, 2004. Available from: http://medschool.mc.vanderbilt.edu/mpb/medphysiology/week2/synapse.III.pdf

Chris M. Wood, C. Louise Milligan, and Patrick J. Walsh, Renal respones of trout to chronic respiriatory and metabolic acidoses and metabolic alkalosis [Internet]. American Journal of Physiology-Regulatory, Intergratiive and Comparative Physiology; Vol. 277, Issue 2, R482-R492, August 1999. Available from: http://ajpregu.physiology.org/cgi/content/full/277/2/R482

Mark T. Worthington, Lauren Browne, Emily H. Battle, and Roger Qi Luo Functional properties of transfected human DMT1 iron transporter [Internet], American Jounral of Physiology-Gastrointestinal and Liver Physiology; Vol. 279, Issue 6, G1265-G1273, December 2000. Available from: http://ajpgi.physiology.org/cgi/content/full/279/6/g125

INDEX

Symptom Index

NOTES

0-595-31499-6